The BIG BOOK of Storysharing

A handbook for personal storytelling with children and young people who have severe communication difficulties

Nicola Grove

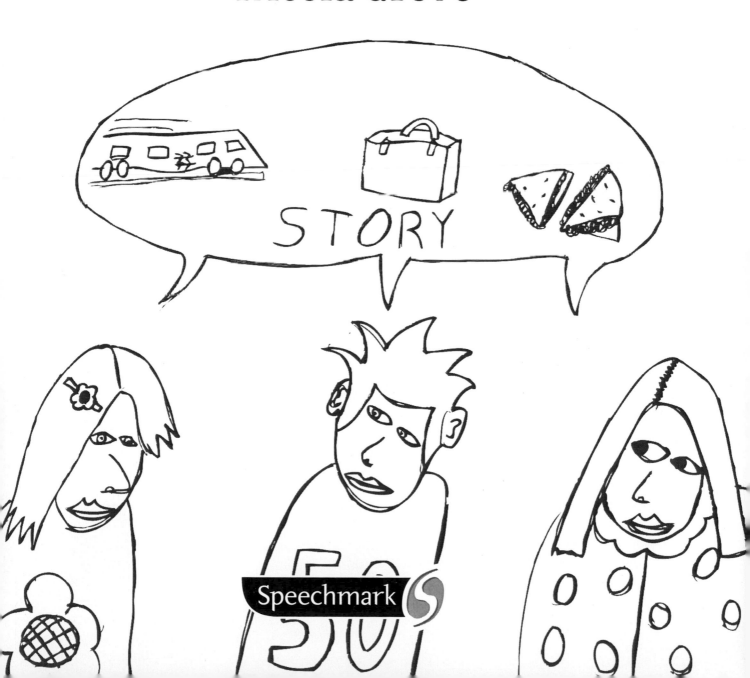

Speechmark

First published in 2014 by
Speechmark Publishing Ltd
St Mark's House, Shepherdess Walk, London N1 7BQ, United Kingdom
www.speechmark.net

© Nicola Grove 2014

Storysharing® is a registered to Openstorytellers Limited.
Openstorytellers are developing certificated training in Storysharing. For details see
www.openstorytellers.org.uk

002-5986 Printed in the United Kingdom by CMP (uk) Ltd
Design and artwork by Moo Creative (Luton)

British Library Cataloguing in Publication Data
A catalogue record for this book is available from the British Library.

ISBN: 978 1 90930 140 5

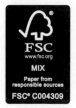

Acknowledgements

This book could not have been written without the ideas and experiences gathered from colleagues, family members, teachers, speech and language therapists, classroom assistants and care workers who have enthusiastically adopted and adapted my original suggestions. Thanks to all of you, and forgive me for not mentioning every single one of you by name. Rosa Morison Day Centre and the Bridge school in London were two of the original sites; Jane Harwood and the team from Openstorytellers have developed and extended projects and training; Woodlands in Harrow, Three Ways in Bath, Critchill and Trinity First in Frome have helped us to implement ideas effectively in school settings. Especial thanks to Nick Peacey and the team at SENJIT, Institute of Education London, who generously funded the first publication. Project funding from various sources is also acknowledged with gratitude: Somerset County Council, Somerset Community Foundation, the Esmée Fairbairn Foundation, the Renton Foundation, London Borough of Harrow, SENJIT, Paul Hamlyn Foundation and the Rayne Foundation. Above all, I express my appreciation of the children and adults with communication difficulties featured here, whose joy in telling stories has provided nonstop motivation and inspiration.

Storysharing is registered to Openstorytellers Ltd. Openstortellers are developing certificated training in Storysharing. For details see www.storytellers.org.uk

Illustrations by Robin Meader, Openstorytellers.

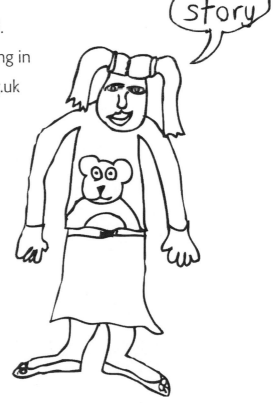

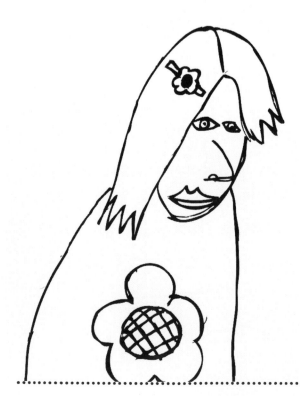

Contents

About this book

This book shows you a way of telling stories with children, so that they can begin to tell stories themselves. It's important to distinguish between telling **to** and telling **with**. You as an adult are there not as the child's instructor, but as the child's friend and partner, and often as their astonished, appalled and delighted audience.

This book has been written to help everyone who comes into contact with children who find it difficult to tell stories independently. They may have special educational needs, or be in the process of learning to speak the language of a new country, or be children who are not used to voicing their experiences and being heard. This method can be used with all of them, because it is a natural approach, based on observations of the ways in which anecdotes are told in everyday life.

Although the book has been written about storytelling with children, you will find that the approach is also useful with adults who have communication difficulties. A report on the implementation of Storysharing® in residential and day centres can be found at **www.openstorytellers.org.uk**.

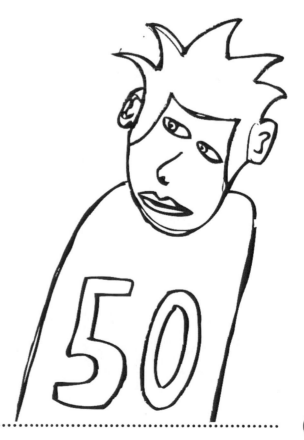

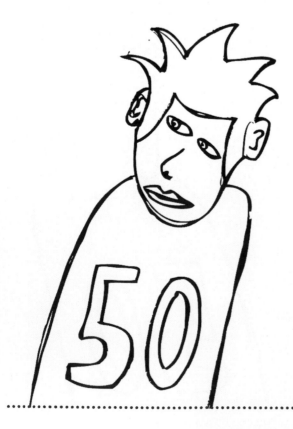

CHAPTER 1

Personal stories we want to share

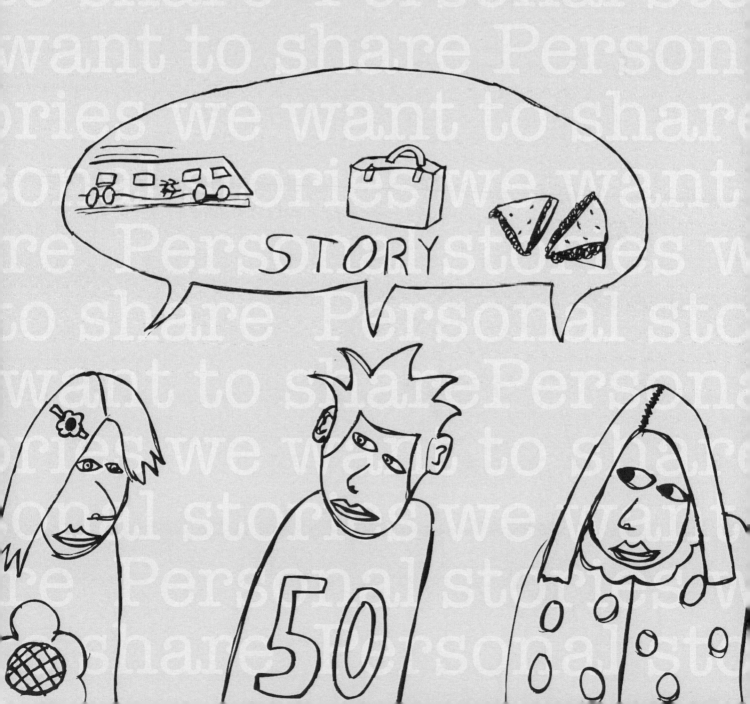

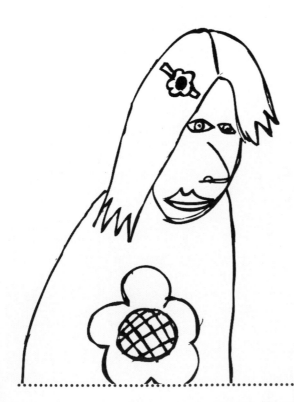

Personal stories in everyday life

First, let's look at a typical story from both adults and children.

Two adults

N: Oh hey, I didn't tell you about my visit to the dentist, did I?

C: No, no you didn't.

N: I'm really, really scared of the dentist …

C: Me too …

N: And so, ever since we moved, I've just stuck with the one I had before, because at least …

C: You know where you are.

N: Exactly, right, exactly. So I went to this one locally, and I mean, it was 50 quid just for a check up …

C: And they don't even do anything then …

N: Yeah, because I'd broken a tooth, so he said I needed to have it crowned, and then he said 'I guess you want to know how much it will cost, don't you?'

C: A lot more than 50 pounds anyway.

N: Yeah, he said it'll be six hundred and eighty-six pounds. (raises her voice) I mean, SIX HUNDRED AND EIGHTY-SIX POUNDS! Mind you, that includes the gas and air, because I am just so, so scared, I just hate the drill, I can't bear it, as soon as I hear that noise …

C: Yeah, I can't stand that. But I bet it would have been more in London.

N: Yeah, well, M said the last time he went, he was quoted a thousand for a crown.

C: It's ridiculous.

N: Yeah, ridiculous. Anyway, I'm just going to have it filled.

This is fairly typical of a conversation between two people who both actively join in the story. The listener (C) is not just giving the feedback that she is listening; she is making her own contributions. The narrative is not a monologue, it is told in spurts, with C on occasions interrupting, both people talking over each other occasionally, and considerable repetition and reinforcement.

Here is another example, with more than two people.

Family narrative

Edith and Ryan (parents), Lucy (9) and Maisie (11) are having lunch with their friends B and N. The conversation turns to the death of the school guinea pigs. N suggests getting a stick insect, but B says this is dull.

Lucy (to N): Well, my insect pet Jennifer, we found her on a basil leaf. And first she was in a little jar, like this, and then we put her in a bigger one, and then a bigger one, and we fed her basil leaves, basil leaves all the time, and she ate them and ate them but then she died. And I wanted to have a funeral, but Mum just threw her away!

Edith: It was rotting! And you weren't doing anything.

Ryan: You should have heard them. The wail that went up. We were in the kitchen and we heard this screaming. Like professional mourners, you know. Ululating, or whatever it is. Unbelievable.

Edith: It appeared on this basil leaf from the supermarket, so we studied it for three days.

Maisie: She shed her skin. We thought she was dying, but she was just shedding her skin.

N: That's fascinating.

Lucy: Yes, we watched her. But then she died anyway.

Maisie (to Edith): And you just chucked her out …

Edith: Well, we did try. We asked if you wanted a funeral, but you said you wanted to do it, but then you just left it. You didn't do anything at all, and then it just rotted and I absolutely didn't want to watch it doing that so I'm afraid I [whish, makes chopping movement with hands].

Lucy: … in the field.

N: Shocking. What unfeeling parents!

Another group narrative

N: So how did it go?

V: We lost the keys there.

N: I don't believe it.

D: Lost the keys and …

V: Oh, did you get your wellies, D?

D: Yes I did.

V: I was leaving …

F: Right.

V: … and I said to D, where can I …

F: … he's not very organised …

D: … no, I'm not.

F: … I did check …

V: …well, that guy did distract us. He was in the room …

F: …said calm down, D, don't worry.

V: We just couldn't' find them, and then, and then – you lost your hearing aid, didn't you D?

D: … my hearing aid, yes. Oh dear, oh dear.

N: Not again. Not AGAIN! Well, at least I know they aren't in MY car …

V: … absolutely, that's just what I said, at least they're not in my car.

N: So we don't have to …

V: …apologise to whatsherface again.

Here again what we see is that in real-life conversations, narratives start, drift, break off, digress, overlap, regain the thread, and make links with previous experiences, acting as the glue to bind a group of friends together. There is an alternation between main narrator and co-narrators, acting as a kind of chorus, more like musical themes and variations than the straight cause and effect reporting that we are accustomed to reading on the page.

Why are personal narratives important?

It has been argued that language emerged out of the need to recount experiences – in other words, to gossip (Dunbar, 1998). Gossip now, of course, is seen as a negative activity, but originally it was a name for your closest female friend. The reason that we need language for telling these personal stories is because we are talking about memories – we can't just point to things or even use simple gestures. We have to use sentences to describe what happened, who was there, and how it felt.

Activity

Think about the last time something eventful happened to you, or to someone you know, from the list below. Can you remember telling the story about it? Can you remember how many times you have told this story?

• An accident

• Losing something important

• Getting annoyed with an official person

• Having a wonderful surprise

• An unexpected encounter

• An amazing coincidence

• Something that made you laugh out loud

You may find that, with a bit of time and space, you can recall an incident for every one of these occasions. You may also start to tell the story again in your head. And you have almost certainly told it on more than one occasion. Actually, we tell these stories quite compulsively, and we actively seek out opportunities to do so when we are with other people. Sitting around with friends, one person starts to talk about their recent holiday and the problems at the airport, and then someone else remembers their last horrendous travel experience and, before you know, it there is a whole chain of tales, until the topic is exhausted and the subject is changed.

Why do we do this? In particular, why do we keep recycling these stories, in situations where our nearest and dearest have already heard them (or perhaps shared in the telling of them) several times already? What do stories do for us?

The value of personal stories seems to lie in the way in which they help us develop a sense of who we are; the role they play in forming and sustaining relationships; the framework they provide for recalling and understanding experience; and the opportunities for imagining possibilities for ourselves that come through hearing the experiences of other people.

Sense of self

If you are asked to describe yourself, or a person you know well, you will probably start with a profile of what you like and don't like, and how you spend your time. This is like a snapshot of you here and now. But actually what may be more significant is how you think of yourself reacting to the experiences you have had. For example, I think of myself as someone who takes on challenges (*positive*) but also as someone who loses things all the time (*negative*), and I have a string of little events in mind to prove each case. In some theories of the self, narrative is seen as absolutely crucial, because our lives follow a narrative path – from birth through growing, seeking out new experiences, and always facing towards the unknown – just like a story, which moves from the past to the present and into the future – which of course is resolved within the story so that a satisfying pattern is completed. Other researchers have written about the way in which we tend to adopt archetypes which are familiar in myths and legends: the hero, the monster, the guide, the mother, the bride. This is, of course, part of the appeal of fictional and traditional stories.

Friendships

Whenever two people meet, you will notice that before long they are sharing anecdotes. Sometimes these are new; often they are reminiscences of times shared together. People can spend whole days in each other's company doing this. Generally, we intersperse the anecdotes with other kinds of conversation: information giving and receiving (where there is no story, but we are catching up on news, or finding out something we need to know to accomplish a task); sharing and responding to each other's mood; deciding together on a course of action (what to eat, where to go). Threaded through these transactions come the anecdotes, as a chance remark sparks a memory. It is hard to imagine sustaining a relationship without the ability to do this. Indeed, we can think of the relationship as having its own identity which is informed not only by shared experience itself, but also by the way we *talk about* that experience.

Recalling and understanding experience

When something happens to us, we appear to be programmed to see it as a narrative. In fact, it is almost impossible to remember any event without it unfolding as a sequence of images in the mind, complete with concepts such as *before, after, when, during, then, and*. Turner (1996), for example, talks about the way we perceive an object falling to the ground as 'a small story in time and space'.

This tendency to see events as unfolding and purposeful seems to be something we are born with (a cognitive predisposition, if you like). It is certainly established through the way we talk about events with other people. This talk helps to embed the memories more firmly: we know, for example, that young children remember events in more detail when they have narrated them out loud.

It also helps us to grasp the meaning of events. When we are faced with an experience which is troubling or perplexing, which we do not quite understand, the act of creating and sharing a narrative about it helps us to make sense of what happened and reassures us, both by giving us control through the way we structure the memory into a familiar form, and through the feedback and empathy we get from others when we tell them about it. Communities do this as well – after important events, whether celebratory or traumatic, people seek out each other to share their experiences, and communal narratives associated with the event are born. Examples might be the tsunami of 2005, '9/11', or Barak Obama's election to the US presidency.

So, to sum up, the ability to tell a personal story helps us to:

- know who we are

- make friends

- remember and understand experience.

As far as we can tell, this kind of storytelling is universal. Even people who do not seem to have any myths or legends in their culture apparently exchange personal anecdotes about their own daily lives (Everett, 2008).

When no stories are told

However, when it comes to children and adults with severe communication and learning difficulties, the picture is very different. Research by Grove (2013) and McHutchison (2006) has shown that, in summary:

- Families and carers find it difficult to recall and tell personal stories from their children's lives.

- Staff tend to share stories with each other, but not with the people they support.

- Services and political initiatives have tended to prioritise choice and individual autonomy over friendships and relationships – so we target requests as our main communication goal.

If we believe that recalling experience and sharing it with others is so fundamental to the ability to develop a sense of self, form relationships and understand our lives, then the implications of never telling stories together are very serious indeed.

The good news is that:

- Everyone can participate in storysharing, regardless of their level of disability.

- Storysharing can lead to improved communication skills, an ability to relate to other people, and an ability to recall events and a stronger sense of community.

Observations

Get yourself a nice notebook to carry around everywhere with you. Start noting down anecdotal conversations. Note not only what is said but also how people move and use gesture, their body language and orientation, their facial expressions, and their tone of voice. Make a note of the ways in which stories are introduced into the conversation and how the teller signals that the story has finished. Note down also what people do when they are listening – again, body language, the responses they make, and the way they move in time with the listener. How do co-narrators work together, and how do they take turns?

In the rest of this book

Storysharing® has been developed over nearly 10 years as an effective narrative tool with both children and adults. This book is your guide, providing the background to the approach, a toolkit for how to do storysharing, how to assess and develop children's skills, and examples from different groups of children with special educational needs. We will be making reference to some different kinds of stories and narratives, so here are some definitions of terms.

Some definitions

anecdote	A short personal account of an event
conversational narrative	Any account of events told as part of a conversation between two or more people
life stories	The autobiographical accounts of the major events in our lives
fictional stories	Any imagined account of events, whether written or told
narrative	An overarching term for all sequenced accounts of events in the order in which they happened
oral narrative/storytelling	Stories which are told face to face. Although the term 'oral' implies that they are always spoken, the signed narrative conversations between deaf people would also qualify here, because they are told in the natural language of the people involved, directly face to face, and are not written down
personal stories	Stories built around individual or group personal experiences
report	An account of events which emphasises the facts
routines	Accounts are often built around routines – ie an accurate description of what usually happens in particular situations, for example at a birthday party, or going to the airport. Routines are predictable
scaffolding	A term used by the Russian psychologist Vygotsky (1978) and others to describe the process through which adults help children to develop their skills by providing just the right amount of support and challenge for them to move forward in learning
script	An account which is repeated in more or less the same way each time, so that it comes to function like a template

social routines	The routines that are involved in social transactions – buying and selling, visiting someone, apologising, complimenting, giving condolences
social stories	A term coined by Carol Gray (www.thegraycenter.org) to describe narratives which help children to understand routines. In the context of Storysharing®, these would not qualify as stories because they are about what usually happens, not about a definite and unexpected event
story	A particular type of narrative, which is always built around an event that is reportable in some way – it is unexpected or notable and therefore worth listening to
traditional stories	Legends, myths and folk tales handed down orally (fairy tales come into this category)
urban myths	Stories which go round groups of people as though they were accounts of something that really happened to someone the speaker has heard of. They relate odd or unusual experiences

Storysharing® and other storytelling approaches

Storytelling is becoming increasingly popular in schools, and there are many other different ways of presenting stories that you may have come across. These may involve:

- telling fictional stories using props or sensory materials

- telling legends and other fictional stories through drama

- helping children to develop the structure of narrative, with the aim of developing literacy

- helping children to make up stories, in drama, for writing down, or for supporting their emotional wellbeing

- developing diaries and pictorial records of things children have done or of their achievements

- digital stories and story apps to create and record stories.

These are all worthwhile and valuable things to do with children. They are not alternatives to Storysharing®; in fact, they can be done alongside, in a complementary way. The conversational technique we use in Storysharing® can be used perfectly appropriately and easily for fictional or invented narratives. The resource list at the end of this book summarises other approaches that you may want to explore.

The key distinguishing features of Storysharing® are:

- stories of personal experience

- told orally (that is face-to-face, dynamically)

- supporting the child as the teller

- a collaborative social model of story.

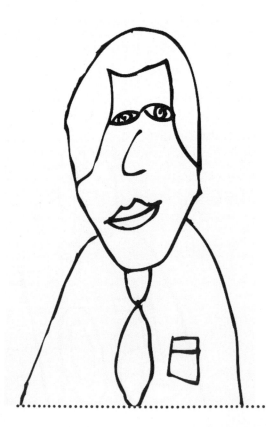

CHAPTER 2

What is a story?

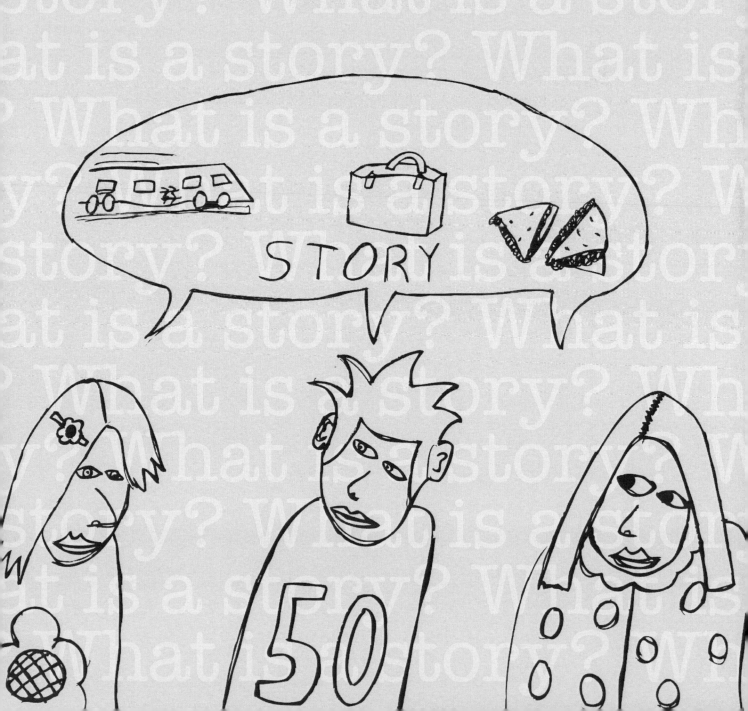

Introduction

When you are trying to identify how to teach a skill to children whose needs are very complex, it is vital to have a clear idea of what you are doing, and how it relates to the strengths and difficulties of the young people concerned.

Storytelling is a very intuitive process that involves many different skills. There are also many different approaches to defining what storytelling (or narrative) is and how best to teach it. We need to think about what kind of stories we are working with, and which approach is best suited to what we are doing. This chapter sets out what we mean by a story and describes some approaches or models of storytelling.

Activity

Complete the following sentence:

A story is …

At the end of this chapter you will find my working definition (it changes from time to time).

Let's start by mapping three different types of narrative.

Type 1 Fictional stories

These cover a range from oral, traditional tales or epics, to literary narratives (novels, etc), to the imaginary monologues that children tell themselves, eg before going to sleep. In their most mature form they are very complex indeed, and associated with a high level of structure. A well-crafted fictional story has:

Characters who face some kind of challenge which has to be resolved, and is part of a network of relationships with other characters. Their motivations and reactions are explored during the story.

Plot which starts with a problem, or an unknown, builds to a climax and ends with a resolution. There are often subplots or diversions from the main plot.

Settings – place and time, well defined with a lot of descriptive language.

The focus in education tends to be on fictional stories composed on the page – oral telling is seen as a way of rehearsing the story before writing it. The main model of narrative which is used for assessment and teaching is sometimes known as *story grammar* because it originates from some work done in the 1970s which suggested that the underlying structure of fictional stories was so predictable and unvarying that it could be thought of as a grammar (ie a structural framework governing the creation of the story)[1]. You have probably come across other sayings about fictional stories such as 'there are only seven kinds of story', or 'all stories have to have a problem'.[2]

Type 2 Personal stories

Sometimes called 'recount narratives', these are the stories that we are focusing on in this book. Personal stories have not been as extensively studied as fictional stories. They tell of our own experiences or those of other people. The context is often conversational, with a social focus on building a sense of relatedness and community. There is a much looser structure, and more collaboration or joining in by listeners. As we have seen from the examples quoted, they can ramble, tail off, morph into different kinds of conversation, start, then deviate, then be picked up again much later on. There seems to be more cultural variation in the way these stories are told than there is in traditional legends[3]. The only real requirement is to hold the attention of the audience, by making sure that the central event is 'reportable'; that is, worth you giving up your valuable time to listen.

The model most used for personal stories comes from researchers who are interested in narratives as a social process – William Labov, Carol Peterson and Alyssa McCabe (Labov, 1972; Labov & Waletzky, 1967; McCabe & Bliss, 2003; McCabe & Peterson, 1991a, 1991b; McCabe *et al*, 2008; Peterson & McCabe 1983; Peterson *et al*, 1999).

Type 3 Accounts and routines

Often when we are asked what happened or what we did, we just give an account of a sequence of events. These accounts are designed simply to put the listener in the picture. They require us to focus (more or less truthfully) on the facts. We may add in some emotion or interest , but we are not required to do so. In some situations (eg witness statements, at the doctor's) we may be actively discouraged from clouding the facts with the feelings. The events we describe may be unique, and they may turn into stories, but the central focus is the facts and information exchange rather than entertainment, social bonding, empathy and sense-making that we discussed in Chapter 1.

Routines are a particular type of account, describing what *usually* happens (eg when we go swimming …). Underlying these narratives is a very powerful structure, which has been called 'generalised event representation' (GER).[4] It's the basic script which allows us to predict what is likely to happen in particular situations. This script is the default setting – and stories are often built on the extent to which what actually happened differed from our expectation of what was going to happen.

Narratives of routines are of interest in special education because they are very useful in helping children with autistic spectrum disorders (ASD) to understand and predict what will occur in the many situations of daily life that they encounter. Carol Gray calls these 'social stories' and she has very helpful guidelines about how to write them (see www.thegraycenter.org). In the context of Storysharing®, these would not count as stories, and it may be easier to think of them as 'social scripts'. Interestingly, of course, it is precisely because the events that feature in stories are unpredictable that storytelling poses some challenges to children with ASD.

The difference between routines and stories is illustrated in Figure 2.1.

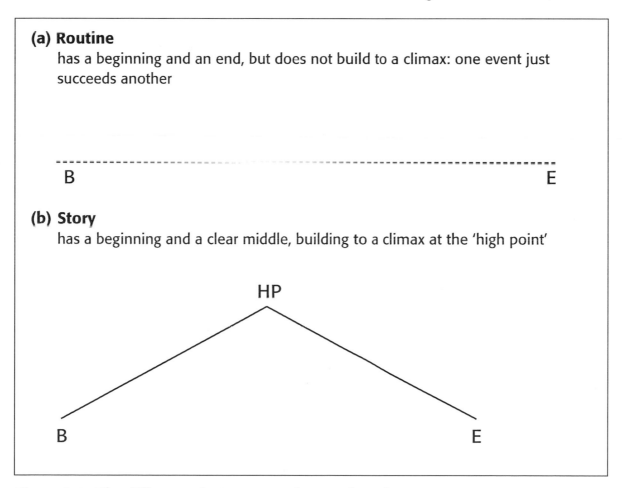

Figure 2.1   The difference between routines and stories

Different approaches to story

Narrative is such a rich area that there are many different definitions and approaches. In education, because the emphasis has been so firmly placed on writing and on fictional stories, the main approach has involved a focus on the structural elements (the *who*, *what*, *where*, *when* and *why*) of the story, and the sequence of events, at the expense of the other aspects of story which are just as important – such as demonstrating feelings, making the story interesting and involving the audience. I call this the 'cognitive approach', because it really is all about cognitive structures and memory, relying heavily on *wh-* questions (often colour coded) as a way of helping children recall a complete story.

When I started storytelling with children with severe learning difficulties, I thought the cognitive approach was the only game in town. I tried really hard to get them to use the *wh-* prompts. We created an exciting event in the classroom, and then we sat down with the children in twos or individually to structure the stories. We used symbol and picture prompts. Then we invited them to sit on a lovely story chair and retell the event, using the prompts. But they just couldn't do it. They couldn't remember, they were shy and they obviously felt put on the spot by being in the chair. I felt a real failure as a teacher.

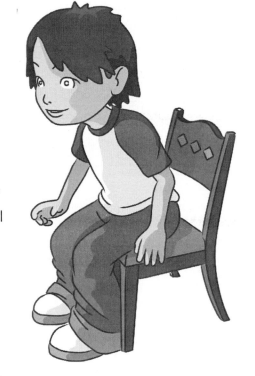

The problem was, I realise now, that we were starting at the wrong end. Given that children are about 5 (mental age) before they confidently include all the *wh-* components (see Chapter 5), it was not really surprising that children with language abilities ranging between about ages 2 and 4 were finding it hard to do. In fact, the story grammar framework on which these prompts are based was originally devised as a way of helping *literate* 7-year-olds with comprehension. One critic of this approach has pointed out that it fails to characterise early child narratives because the focus is always on what they are leaving out or *not* doing (Nicolopoulou, 1997).

So I had to throw away the book and start again. What we ended up with was group retelling, led at first by myself or one of the teachers or speech therapy students (thank you Alison and Louise). We went overboard on the acting, using exaggerated tones of voice, lots of gesture and some signs, and lots of dramatic pauses. I found myself using one phrase over and over again: 'AND THEN …!' The children picked up on this and started to say and sign it to link the events. They joined in with what they could remember. There was no pressure and, freed from the terror of The Chair, they just started relaxing and enjoying the story.

When I read around narrative to see if I could find any theoretical or evidence-based justification for the methods I had developed through trial and (lots of) error, I realised that I had inadvertently bought into a different approach: the social model of storytelling. The social model was developed through the study of personal narratives, and puts an equal emphasis on the feelings and audience involvement to that on the structure of the story; and it regards narrative development as a social process which begins in infancy and is scaffolded by adults. Appendix 1 provides a comparison between cognitive and social approaches.

So the first message is that if you are working with children who are developmentally delayed, and operating below an age equivalent to about 4, you might find that the social model works better than the cognitive model, because it tells us more about very early narrative and places more emphasis on what interactive partners are doing. For children with profound disabilities, you simply can't operate a cognitive approach, but the social approach offers a number of possibilities.

I should say, however, that there are many therapists and teachers out there who are using *wh-* prompts really successfully with preschool children – so it may work very well for you. The important thing is to know which model is appropriate in which situations. The social model offers advantages when working with different cultures, if your target is emotional literacy, and if you are working on personal stories. The cognitive model is more suited to highly structured fictional narratives which will be written down. A range of approaches are described in Grove (2013), including sensory storytelling, call and response storytelling, and tactile books.

Choose your focus

Working with different cultures

A difficulty with the dominant cognitive model is that it was developed on the basis of East European folk tales and a very particular white, western way of narrating. There is now quite a body of research that demonstrates that oral telling is very culturally determined (and I suggest that this is even more pronounced with personal narratives). To summarise, comparative research on narratives from different ethnic groups in the USA (see Dickinson, 1991; Gutierrez & Quinn, 1993; and the extended discussion in McCabe & Bliss, 2003) suggests that:

- Japanese children told stories that were succinct, focused on the main event, and were not elaborated or strongly evaluated
- children from Hispanic backgrounds emphasised personal networks and relationships
- children from African-Caribbean backgrounds strongly evaluated and dramatised their narratives.

Worryingly, researchers found not only that children were being taught to conform to the dominant narrative (middle-class white European), but also that they were actually being marked down because their narratives were thought to be inadequate (Hispanic and African-Caribbean children too talkative and Japanese children not talkative enough). Clearly, the teachers were profoundly ignorant of the cultural traditions that the children were bringing with them into the classroom. This affects children with special educational needs as well as typically developing children – I was interested to see that a child with language and communication difficulties who was telling a halting story in English used a traditional ending from her own culture (Pashtun) which her support teacher happily recognised.

Because the social model focuses on the context of narrative, there is less structural prescription about the way the narrative is told, and more room for including culturally appropriate scaffolding. You should always try to find out as much as possible about the way in which personal narratives are shared in the child's own culture (although this can be difficult as there is not a lot of research to go on, and people may find it hard to consciously analyse what they are doing).

Working with emotional literacy

Perhaps the greatest argument in favour of the social model is that it places such an emphasis on the meaning of the story and its emotional significance to teller and listener and the way that is conveyed to the audience. By contrast, the cognitive model has almost nothing to say about meaning. Labov once trenchantly remarked that a story which consisted only of structural elements was nothing more than a list (quoted in Fox, 1993).

In Storysharing® we start with the expression of feelings and the build-up to the climax. Feelings offer the key to the story – we tell other people about events that have generated some kind of emotional response in us, be that anger, amusement, excitement or fear. We also focus on listening, empathy and response in the audience, which is as important as the telling.

Working with personal narratives

Oral, anecdotal narratives are less structurally demanding than fictional narratives because they can be interesting without needing complex plots (Hudson & Shapiro, 1991; McCabe *et al*, 2008). Linguistically, they can be told with very simple linkage – *and, then, so.* Because they rely on a lot of emotional expression and nonverbal strategies, the social model captures more of their essence than the cognitive model. Personal narratives are a really good way to start storytelling.

Working with fictional narratives

If your focus is clearly on constructing an imaginative story with a plot and characters in a particular setting, with children who are mature enough to be including these elements at least sometimes in their oral narratives, then the cognitive model works very well. However, I think it is important not to push children too quickly into complex linguistic constructions. Some of our greatest literature (the Bible, Homer) uses very simple sentences linked by 'and' to great literary effect.[5]

The Storysharing® definition

The framework that we have developed, over the past 10 years in Openstorytellers, is based on the social model, but is also informed by other researchers who have emphasised the pragmatic, cultural conventions, and the poetic patterning of oral narrative – rhythmic riffs, pitch changes and repetitions.[6]

Definition of story
A story is a representation of a reportable experience, associated with a strong feeling, that we want to share with another person.

How did this working definition compare with yours at the start of the chapter? There is quite a lot left out of it – for example, I haven't included the structural elements like a beginning, an end and ordering. This is because I like to think that these elements are implicit in the representation of the experience. But we could add them in:

A story is shared with other people in the form of a narrative with a beginning, middle and end.

The centre is the reportable experience, which generates a feeling, which motivates us to gain the attention of a listener, and to engage in a story interaction or conversation.[7]

Analysing the skills of telling a story

Now we've defined what a story is, we need to identify what skills are involved in telling it.

Activity

Watch someone telling a personal story. Make a list of the skills that you notice the person is using.

If we think through what actually happens in the telling of a story, we can identify the following components that need to be in place.

1 Audience awareness

We have to be aware of the listener and how to get and sustain interest, and how to signal that we have finished. This is the pragmatics of storytelling, what we might call 'audience awareness'. It includes beginnings and endings as well as some nonverbal behaviours such as eye contact, body orientation and gestures.

2 Emotional expression and perspective

Right from the start, the teller conveys how she or he feels about the event and an expectation of what the listener's response should be. These feelings are conveyed through body language, gesture, tone of voice and facial expressions, as well as the words we choose to use: *disgusted, delighted, really really bad, just fantastic*. So these feeling aspects are both verbal and nonverbal. Labov (1972) calls these elements 'evaluations' because they tell the listener how to judge (evaluate) the experience.

3 Structural

Of course, we are also going to look at how the child manages the structural elements: the *who, when, where, what happened, how* and *why* of story, as well as the logical sequencing, causal links and how accurately and fully the events are recalled.

4 Language

We look for the way the child uses language: vocabulary and sentence structure. You need verbs and adjectives to tell a story well, and specific nouns. (One lady I know well finds it really hard to get at the specific names for things and is always talking about 'the whatsit' and 'the whosit', which makes it really difficult to follow what she is wanting to tell me.)

Interestingly, in oral personal narratives you don't always need verb tenses, since the present tense is so often used (you don't need it in sign language narrative either), and you can get away with a simple time marker. Some linking words (*and, then, so* and later *because)* are very useful.

5 Patterning and poetry

Lastly, we are interested in the way the story works almost as a musical composition – the patterns, rhythms, tones and phrasing – as well as the way in which they deploy culturally specific narrative conventions (you see more of these in traditional fictional stories, but they do sometimes seep into conversational telling). In this category I put repetition, well-known phrases, sayings and clichés, the riffs and strophes that give the oral narrative its poetic, cultural and personal identity

Summary

A story is centred on a 'reportable' experience, that is, one that is worth the telling: memorable because it is a departure from what we expect (the generalised event with its defined script) – and the feeling that this generates. When we come to share our memory with another person, we organise the telling in five key dimensions:

- audience awareness
- feelings and perspectives
- structure and cognition
- language
- patterning and poetry.

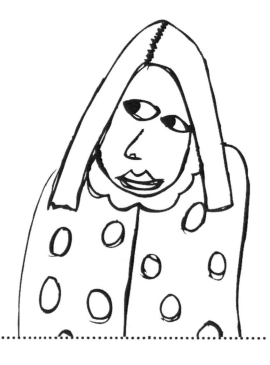

Notes

1   'Story grammar' was a term used by Rumelhart in 1975, and Mandler & Johnson in 1977, as a way of capturing the fact that many fictional stories seemed to have a predictable underlying structure, first analysed in *Morphology of the Folktale* by Vladimir Propp in the 1920s. The main aim of story grammar is explicitly to help children develop cognitive literacy, through working on reading comprehension. A good overview is provided by Stein & Albro (1997).

2   The notion of seven stories was taken up by Christopher Booker (2004) in his book *The Seven Basic Plots*. Propp's analysis of folk tales demonstrated that they usually involve a problem or challenge, and this has been generalised to other story types. It is very common to find statements such as 'most stories start with a problem or challenge that the hero must resolve', and it is a short step from this to saying that a story *has* to have a problem.

3   Fiestas & Pena (2004) found that children in classrooms in the USA who had come from Central America had more exposure to conversational than to literary narratives, and hence less experience with the educationally privileged narrative structure emphasising events, problems, cause and effect than children from European backgrounds.

4   A full account of GERs can be found in Nelson & Gruendel (1986).

5   For example, 'And they heard the voice of the Lord God walking in the garden in the cool of the day. And Adam and his wife hid themselves from the presence of the Lord God amongst the trees of the garden. And the Lord God called unto Adam and said to him, Where art thou? And he said, I heard thy voice in the garden and I was afraid because I was naked and I hid myself' (Genesis 3: 8–10). The linking 'and' is regarded as 'primitive' in some models, but in this epic text you can see its very simplicity is essential for the dramatic effect.

6   Hymes (1981) calls this the ethnopoetics of narrative; Norrick (2000) found that these rhetorical devices played a key role in conversational anecdotes.

7   Labov & Waletzky (1967), developed by Peterson & McCabe (1983) in their research with young children.

CHAPTER 3

How to develop a story

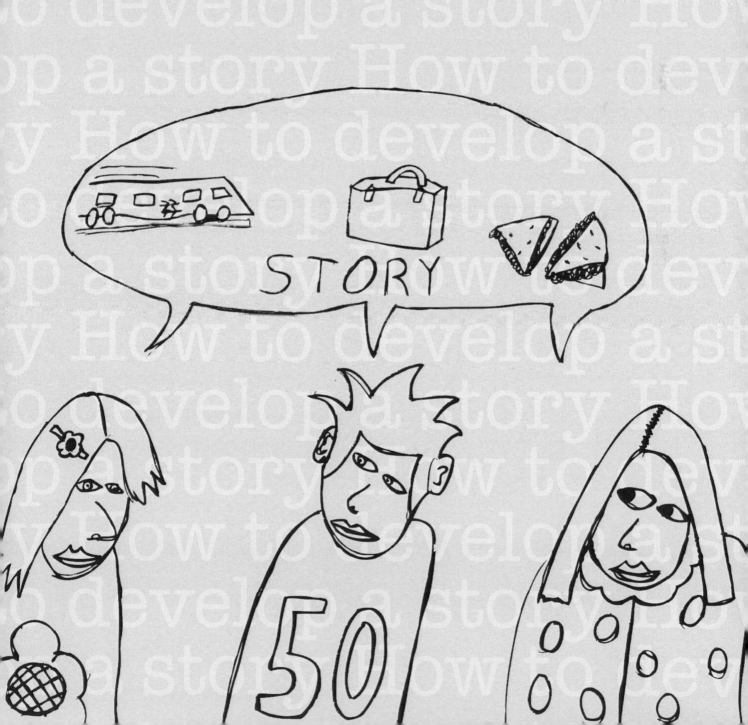

Introduction

Telling stories about our experiences is so natural to us that we may not recognise just how much goes into it. We have to differentiate between the process of identifying and constructing the story (Stage 1) and actually telling the story (Stage 2).

In this chapter we will look at: how to recognise a reportable experience, how to remember it and how to make it into a story – Stage 1 of the process of Storysharing®.

Remember how we are defining a story:
- a representation
- of a reportable experience
- that generates a feeling
- and that we want to share with others.

It follows then that in order to create a good story, we need to have:
- an experience that can be made into a story
- a memory (representation) of that experience that we draw on
- the motivation to tell it – generated by our feelings
- a willing and responsive audience.

The experience

In Chapter 2, I argued that we do not, generally, make stories out of predictable, routine experiences. Rather, we store up the little excursions from the norm that are interesting and worth narrating. In the social model, stories always have a 'high point' or climax, around which the expression of feelings clusters:

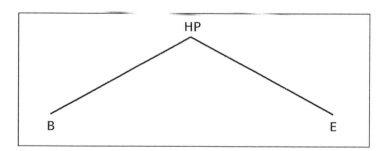

So we generally remember the event that started the story (B), the climax (HP), and then how the story ended (E) – usually about three episodes.

Reportable experiences can be very dramatic – one participant on a course related how she had been robbed at gunpoint – but they can also be very trivial indeed: momentarily forgetting where you parked your car; an irritating phone call; finding something you had just mislaid – just as long as there is something that makes the event stand out in our minds.

The feelings

What makes the event stand out is the association with an emotional reaction, whether positive or negative.

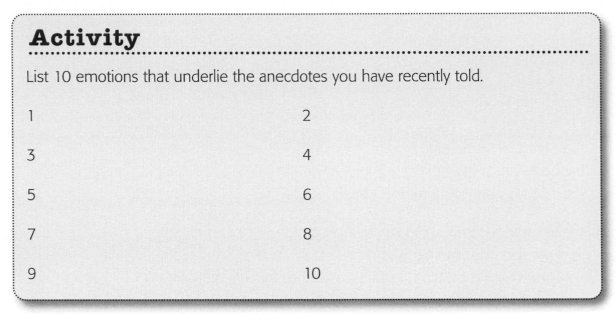

Activity

List 10 emotions that underlie the anecdotes you have recently told.

1   2

3   4

5   6

7   8

9   10

Figure 3.1 List of emotions that are commonly involved in everyday storytelling.

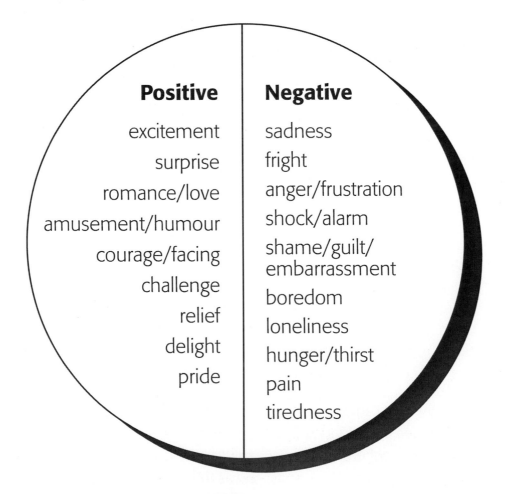

Positive	Negative
excitement	sadness
surprise	fright
romance/love	anger/frustration
amusement/humour	shock/alarm
courage/facing	shame/guilt/embarrassment
challenge	boredom
relief	loneliness
delight	hunger/thirst
pride	pain
	tiredness

Figure 3.1 Common emotions in storytelling

It is noticeable that we tell stories more about negative than positive emotions,[8] and this is certainly true of children's early narratives, which often revolve around accidents or illness. This, of course, has quite profound implications for the experiences that (a) we allow children to have and recall and, (b) we allow them to share with others. Generally, we try to protect our children who have special educational needs from negative experiences and to minimise their impact. There are sometimes ethical complications and risks involved in creating or recalling reportable experiences (see 'Troubleshooting' in Chapter 5).

The memory

Activity

Shut your eyes and call up a memory of the last story you told.
• What is that memory composed of?
• What goes into it?

We can think of a memory as a collection of sensory representations.

The most obvious or dominant is probably the **visual** images: what we can see in our mind's eye – not only the background details of the place, and our image of the people, but also watching the events unfold.

Another critical sense is **hearing** – we can often call up the sounds associated with the event. We tend to think of background noise, but actually the most important sounds in anecdotal telling are what people said – the tone of voice as well as the actual words.

Movement, **touch**, **smell** and **taste** are, of course, other powerful sensory representations. However, there is a difference between the ways vision and hearing work in memory compared with these more primitive senses. Generally, you can call up visual and to some extent auditory images to order. However, it is much more difficult to consciously recall taste, smell, touch and movements. For example, I can remember sliding on an icy pond when I was a small girl. I can see the park and my blue snowsuit. If I work really hard, I can just about remember my mother's voice telling me to be careful. But I can't actually *feel* the cold, or myself sliding. Nor can I *taste* the snow that I licked.

These basal or proximal senses are processed in the part of the brain which is not accessible to conscious recall. However, as we know, the process works powerfully the other way – when you smell or taste something from your past that was associated with a significant event, you immediately recall the visual and auditory images as well. We have to be quite careful about how we use these proximal sensory inputs, because they are very powerful and persistent – it's not a good idea to use too many contrasting smells and tastes within one story.

Memory can be helped by the use of:

- a key object, such as an object of reference, which you bring away as a memento. For example: a bunch of keys for the lost key story; a torn shopping bag for the bag that bursts; a chocolate wrapper for finding what I like. Be careful, however, not to overload the story with props, or the task becomes one of handling objects rather than remembering and telling the story

- a simple communication aid, such as a Big Mack®, which you can immediately record responses and reactions on.

Motivation

So, once we have had an experience that has generated a powerful memory and feelings, we think about sharing it. We want to do this for different reasons, as discussed in Chapter 1, and our motives can be very complex:

- to entertain
- to relieve our own feelings
- to build empathy
- to get support
- to make sense of what has happened
- to help us remember better.

On their own, though, these understandable reasons do not quite explain the very human phenomenon of repeating a story we have already told (often to the same audience!). We are always recycling our anecdotes. Maybe this is something to do with the patterned and musical structure involved. The one certainty in our lives is that we are moving towards the unknown. We never get to finish and look back on our life stories. However, when we tell and retell a story, we are completing a pattern for ourselves. The closure and resolution of a story is enormously satisfying. This means that we need to pay attention to the underlying rhythmic structure of the story, like with a musical composition.

The audience

What makes a receptive audience? You need people who are willing to listen, to respond, and to give you their full attention. When we focus on listening with children, it is usually in a context where we want them to take in and remember information. So we emphasise sitting still and quiet, with 'ears open, mouths shut, eyes looking'. Actually listening to anecdotes involves rather different behaviour – very active body language and 'mirroring' of the speaker, lots of animated feedback that signals how you feel about their story, and which acts to motivate the speaker to continue. Often, as we have seen, it will involve joining in, finishing sentences, or taking over the narration.

Another relevant issue is whether the listener already knows the story. Research shows that stories are told more fully to new listeners (Liles, 1993) So the ideal audience will include at least one person who has not heard the story before. Listeners who are 'in the know', have to play the game by not spoiling the story, demonstrating interest – and will sometimes join in and contribute, depending on their relationship with the teller. You may need to teach the other children in the class how to be responsive listeners (see Chapter 5, 'Storysharing® in practice').

You also need time and space to tell your story. Anecdotes can actually be shared quite quickly – during a journey, waiting for a bus, attending to personal care needs are all times when you can enjoy a simple memory together. At other points we can take an extended period to gossip and exchange our stories, as a group or with one other person, often when our hands are occupied with another task such as clearing up, having a drink, driving, looking at photos together.

In terms of *spaces*, the environment needs to be quiet enough to hear each other. Sitting in circles or semicircles allows everyone to see each other, and the space between you, which is where the story happens, needs to be intimate enough for the exchange, but not so close that the story cannot move and breathe. You need as well to be able to focus on each other for the best exchange of stories. Although it may be very helpful and enjoyable for children to look at pictures of the story on a whiteboard, it's not a good space for actually telling the story to each other, as attention then has to be split – and inevitably the pictures will dominate.

So, to summarise, in order to create a story, a child needs:

- a reportable experience
- a representation of that experience
- feelings and a means of expression
- a reason to share the experience
- an audience.

Putting the principles into practice

Find the experience for the child

You will either be in the position of creating the experience, making the most of an experience which just happens, or recalling with the child an experience that someone has told you about.

Experiences as they happen

Once you are on the look out, reportable experiences happen all the time. What you need to do is to draw the child's attention to them, and then make the space to retell them, ideally straight away. Mostly we brush these aside and focus on the important things we need to engage with – the lesson, lunch, getting home. Of course, you can't always drop everything and pay attention to the event – but do so if possible.

Experiences you are told about

Try to get as much information as you can from the informants, including the child if possible. This means asking about all the sensory inputs: where it happened, what the child saw and heard – not forgetting what people said, any smells, tastes and movements you could include. The best way is to encourage your verbal informants to tell you the story themselves, and if possible record them. You can then follow up with probe questions. If this isn't possible, your main method is to ask direct questions about who, when, where, what happened, how it felt, what was said. You can ask carers, siblings, staff, friends and the children themselves. We use the structure set out in the record form (see Appendix 2). It is really important to try to get down verbatim what people said at the time (remember that voice and recorded speech is the medium of anecdotal story).

Creating the experience

It is all too common to find that no one can remember anything noteworthy in the child's life – in which case you can always create an unexpected event.

Lose your keys and get the children to hunt round the classroom; make a cake and drop it on the floor as it comes out of the oven (and don't produce one you made earlier, follow an event through to its natural consequence); bring in a dog; spill paint all over the table; arrange for a surprise parcel to be delivered.

Developing memory

If you want the child to recall the event, you need to make it possible for them to attend to the event. This means that they must have the opportunity to process at least something of what is going on. While the event is happening, try to help the children by:

- drawing their attention to the experience – use all the tactile, sound and smell cues available at the time (eg in a visit to a garden centre; flowers, the feel of wet leaves on their cheek, wind blowing, feel of vegetables pulled from the ground, earth on their hands)

- collecting a memento to put in a story box or scrapbook. Give it to the child to take charge of and look after on the way home

- reacting very strongly yourself – laughing, exclaiming, smacking your forehead, and repeating this over and over again

- using a 'refrain' – something people say in reaction to what happens that you can repeat over and over again: 'Oh my goodness', 'You look great!', 'What on Earth?' You will use these same cues when you retell the story. Try also to record what the child does at the time, and refer to this in the retelling.

By all means take a digital photo or a short video clip – but this should be used only as a prompt for the story, not as a substitute for telling it.

As the story will be conveyed through words and voice, emphasise key words and intonation. Name the feelings – both how you feel and how you think the child is reacting. Record the story on a simple form (see Appendix 2 and Figure 3.2).

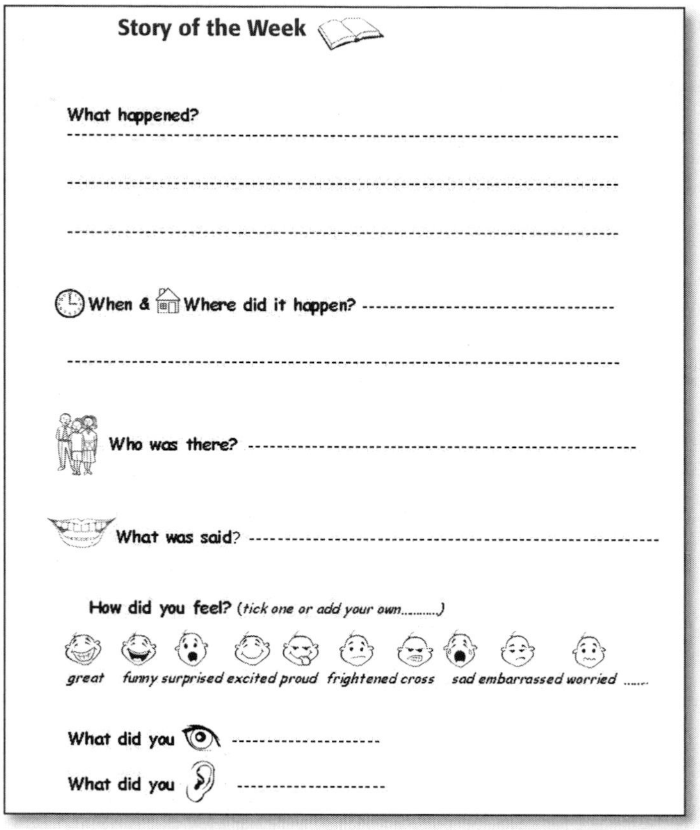

Story of the Week

What happened? --

When & Where did it happen? --

Who was there? --

What was said? --

How did you feel? (*tick one or add your own..........*)

great funny surprised excited proud frightened cross sad embarrassed worried ......

What did you ------------------

What did you ------------------

Figure 3.2 Example of a story form

Record the story

Immediately after we have had a reportable experience, we start to structure it in the form of a story. This often means that we go over it in our minds, mentally selecting some bits, discarding others. Children with special needs are unlikely to be able to do this independently, so you need to support them.

1 Let them know the experience was reportable: 'That was **so** awful. But you were really brave'/'That was so funny, I've never seen you laugh so much'.

2 Let them know that the story is worth telling to someone else: 'I really think that mum/Miss White/the class ought to hear this story'.

3 Structure it: 'Let's see if we can remember what happened'. Here you can start to prompt, use photos or pictures if you have them, use key objects of reference.

4 Make an accessible record of the story.

There are lots of ways of recording stories. One is to have a scrapbook with the story on one side and a memento on the other. Another way is to have a coloured envelope in which you put the small object. Mementoes can be anything that is collected at the time of the event (Musselwhite, 1990):

• a parking ticket

• a leaf

• a paper napkin from a café

• a key (one you don't use, obviously).

Depending on the story:

• a story box with objects and the story on a card

• a story bag.

After a lot of experimentation, we came up with a form we use for recording stories (see Figure 3.2). This provides the key information in a very simple form.

You want to avoid writing out the whole story in diary form. Although this is tempting, we have found that once teachers do this, the story gets read rather than told, and all the repetitions and pauses and intonation that are characteristic of orally told anecdotes get edited out.

Activity

Devise your own record form for capturing the key elements of an event that you think would make a good story.

Now make your own story book, bag or box.

Summary

In this chapter we have identified:

- the nature of story memory

- the steps involved in making an experience reportable and memorable

- how to record a story.

We will now move on to the next stage, which is how to share the story.

Notes

8 Hudson *et al* (1992) found that stories about positive events, evoking happiness, were more focused on mood than on dynamic action, whereas negative (angry or scary) stories were more likely to be centred on a high point. In our work, we found the same thing – stories about a nice trip out, a birthday or a picnic meander, and just evoke the response, 'Ooh, lovely …'.

CHAPTER 4

How to share a story

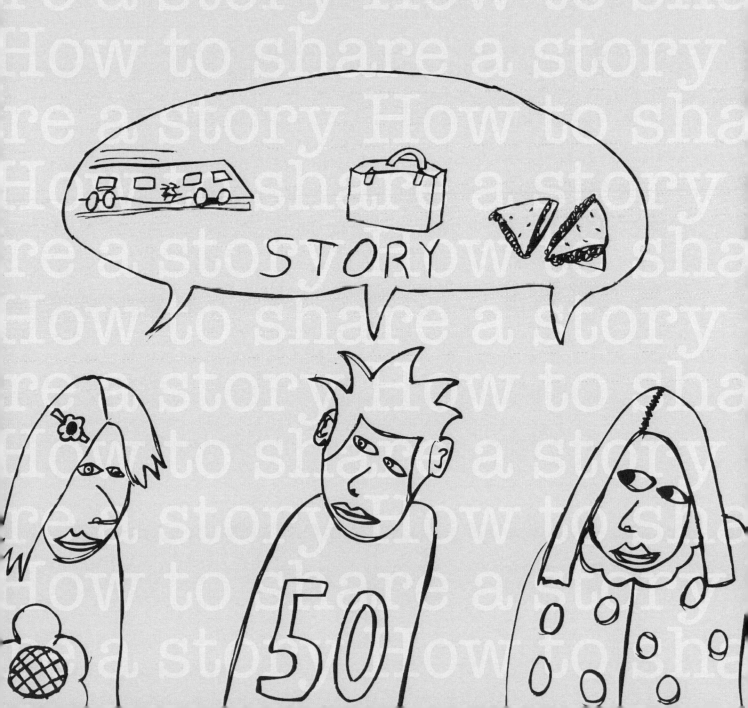

Introduction

Once we have identified the experience to be made into a story, we need to think about how to support the child to tell it. This chapter deals with Stage 2 of Storysharing® – joint telling and the conversational techniques to support it.

Asking what happened and telling what happened

In daily life with children and adults who do not have communication difficulties, if you ask what happened it is often enough to elicit a full anecdotal narrative. But with young children and with children who have special needs, the process of finding out the facts of the story and narrating the story get conflated. Typically, adults start by asking what happened, get some answers from the child and stop at this point. They think the story has been told. But it hasn't. All that has happened is that you have found out the facts behind the story. How often have you heard the following kind of exchange?

(A = adult, C = child)

A: *Tell Nicola about what you did yesterday.*

C: *[Looks at the floor. Silence.]*

A: *Where did we go?*

C: *Playground.*

A: *What did we do there?*

C: *Swings.*

A: *Yes, we went on the swings. And what happened after we were on the swings? Tell Nicola.*

C: *[Silence.]*

A: *Do you remember? We saw something didn't we? What did we see?*

C: *[Silence.]*

A: *Did we see a dog or a cat?*

C: *Cat.*

A: *No, we didn't see a cat, did we? We saw a dog, didn't we?*

C: *Dog.*

A: *Yes that's right, a dog. And what did the dog do?*

C: *[Silence.]*

A: What did the dog do? Do you remember?

C: [Silence.]

A: It jumped up, didn't it? And got us all muddy.

C: Muddy.

A: Muddy, that's right. And what did you do?

C: [Silence.]

A: You laughed, didn't you?

This is not telling a story. It's an interview. The child is put on the spot, and prefers to remain silent rather than risk a wrong answer, whether or not she actually remembers. If you try this yourself as a role play you will feel how pressurising it is to be asked a series of direct questions. As an interviewer, the problem with these direct questions is that it drives both of us into a cul-de-sac. We have nowhere to go. The child can either give the right answer, the wrong answer, or remain silent. But if we don't get the answer we expect, we also start to panic slightly, and our principal strategy seems to be to ask a yes/no, or a 'forced alternative' question (dog or cat). Both of these question types lay traps.

People who are disempowered in conversation tend to give affirmative answers (*acquiescence bias*; see Heal & Sigelman, 1995), and are unlikely to deny or assert the contrary. So even if you try to provoke them by asking a question they know to be false (eg 'Did we see an elephant?'), they may answer 'Yes', which means you then have to correct them, reinforcing their sense of uncertainty and disempowerment.

With forced alternative questions, we know that children and adults with processing difficulties tend to echo the last word they hear (the *recency effect*: see Baddeley, 1997). If you give them the wrong alternative last, they will simply repeat it.

Instead of looking at the child's responses as negatives, let's examine what she actually does in this conversation.

• She clearly remembers where they went and what they did.

• She can give one-word answers

• She can imitate what is said.

• She stays with the conversation and doesn't get up and leave.

So we need to build on these skills, and find a way of enabling her to take the initiative in telling her story

Observation

Activity

Sit and listen to people in conversation with a young child and a child with special needs. Note how often questions are used, and the response to the questions.
- What other strategies do adults use?
- Which seem to be the most effective?

Preparation

Ideally, you and the child will rehearse the story together, using the record that you made together as a basis. Telling a story is like putting on a small performance. The child knows that you know about the story – so there is no anxiety about failure, as you are there as the safety net. The point is *not* to **find out** what happened; it is to **tell** someone what happened. We do this by letting the child know what a significant event this is, and what a good story it makes.

We go through the story record with the child, prompting, helping their memory by whatever means. We decide together if there is an object or a picture which could be used in the story. We act out bits of the story, and demonstrate how to show feelings, modelling them, sitting side by side with the child and encouraging imitation and echoing. We are looking for the contributions that the child can make, independently or with help, to the story. Once we have established together what happened, we put the story record away, and concentrate on rehearsing how we are going to tell it.

Activity

Think of a nonverbal child who you know well.
List the things that he or she could do to take part in a story.

You should have come up with some or all of the following:

- vocalise to communicate a feeling
- vocalise to communicate a sound (eg animal noise, wind blowing, person panting)
- use body to make sounds – eg footsteps, clapping
- press a voice output communication aid to make a sound
- use an instrument – eg drum, bells, shaker
- show an object or a picture
- communicate feelings through body language
- communicate feelings through facial expression
- join in with other people's sounds and speech
- imitate a word or sound
- perform an action
- use a gesture
- eye point to indicate a person, place or thing in the story
- point or reach using hands to indicate a person, place or thing in the story.

So in the rehearsal, you and the child identify together what he or she will do and what you will do to join in the story. Let the child know how brilliant her contribution is. Foreground it as you tell it by dramatically pausing as you hand over to the child. Prompt wherever necessary: prompting is all part of the process. If you do not have the time for a specific practice session, you can do quick short rehearsals just before you tell the story – identifying one thing that the child will do to contribute, and practising that bit.

Your aim is to keep the narrative 'balloon' up in the air, moving between you and the child (Figure 4.1). Do this by constructing the narrative thread yourself and allow the child to add 'beads' rather than by a question and answer routine. Storysharing is the name we give to this process.

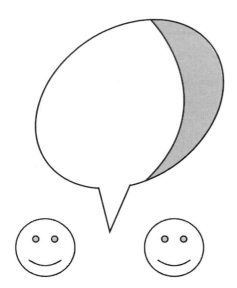

Figure 4.1 The Storysharing balloon

The child inputs part of the story (shaded) and you do the rest

The Storysharing® technique

The basic Storysharing® technique involves three conversational strategies.

Minimise direct questions. People find this incredibly difficult to do. When you are starting out with sharing stories, you should actually aim for *no* direct questions. As you get more comfortable with the technique, you will find you can slip in the odd question that does not seem confrontational, and will allow the child to respond.

Use sentence completion. You start the sentence, and leave a gap for the child to join in. If you have done your observations of natural anecdotes, you will have realised how often we do this anyway.

Use 'and then …' as a linking device. To lead into the child's contribution, say *'and then…'* and leave a dramatic pause. We have found that most children find this an irresistible stimulus to take part.

Another linking strategy is 'like …', which is a signal that the teller is going to move into dramatic or nonverbal mode. *'And she's, like, I am so not going there'*; *'And I'm, like, derrr!'.* This is a very powerful way of handing over. You say *'and you were, like …',* pause, hand over, so that it is the child who shows the facial expression, makes the sound, or provides the reported speech on a voice output device.[9]

So, for example, the playground conversation earlier, reconfigured as sharing the story, would go something like this.

A: Let's tell Nicola about what happened to us yesterday. Nicola, you just won't believe what happened to Sharon. We went to the p ...

C: Playground.

A: And when we were in the playground you were playing on the ...

C: Swings.

A: And then all of a sudden, all of a sudden, we were just playing and we heard this really loud barking and it was a d ...

C: Dog.

A: This big dog, which came running up, and I was a bit scared, I don't mind telling you, but Sharon, Sharon was amazing, she just stood there, and this dog, this dog you'll never guess what it did, it j ...

C: Jumped up!

A: Yeah, jumped up, like this [A and C mime dog jumping up], and then ...

C: Fell over (laughs).

A: She fell over! And like I was so cross with the dog owner, I shouted 'Get your dog off ! Can't you control your dog!' And the guy ran up and he was saying, he was saying – let's press the Big Mack[10] to show Nicola.

C: [Presses Big Mack] 'I'm so sorry.'

A: But Sharon, Sharon was amazing, she was incredibly brave, she was like –

C: Laughing!

A: She was laughing. You thought it was really really f ...

C: Funny!

A: But I said to the guy, 'Well it was OK this time but you really really need to be careful with that dog.' But Sharon gave the dog a pat and then it ...

C: Licked me!

A: Yeah, licked her face. With its tongue. Sharon will show you!

C: [Sticks out her tongue.]

The advantage of this technique is that you have a number of options if the child remains silent or says the wrong thing. Basically, you work up a prompting hierarchy, from the full gap to a full word or sign.

Prompting levels

Level 1 Full gap

You start the sentence and leave a gap to be completed by the child, either with a word or a sign or a gesture:

We went to the …

You can also sign as a prompt. A manual sign that the child knows well will often elicit the spoken word automatically.

Level 2 Initial sound

We went to the p …

And/or initial sign:

Hold the handshape and location of the sign within the child's vision.

Level 3 Partial words

We went to the play …

We went to the playgr …

And/or partial signs:

Make the sign action briefly, hold it and wait for the child to join in.

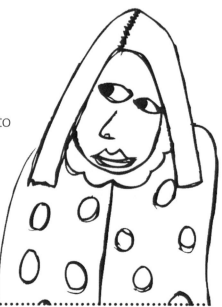

Level 4 Full word and sign prompt

We went to the [pause] playground.

And/or prompt the child's hands, or encourage her to put her hands on yours as you make the sign.

Then you drop your hands so that she is making the sign herself.

Always reinforce the child's contribution and carry on:

Yeah, so Sharon and I went to the playground (great signing, Sharon).

Repetition

Repeating what the child has said is a really natural way of furthering the dialogue. If you listen to stories being told, you will notice how often people repeat themselves and each other. You can repeat almost as many times as you like, since anecdotal conversation is riddled with repetitions and echoes of what has previously been said. The repetitions initially confirm what the child has said (implicitly valuing it), help the child to recall the information, and buy the child time to remember what happens next.

Sharon will tell you with me where we went.

Level 1

We went to the …

[Child does not respond so adult says] Playground.

Level 2

Yeah, we went to the p …

[Child does not respond, so adult continues.]

The playground is amazing at this time of year, it's got so many lovely flowers.

Level 3

So we went to the playgr…

[Child does not respond, adult carries on.]

We go there a lot, but this time something happened. So yesterday, there we were in the …

[Sign PLAYGROUND with the child]

…the playground, good signing, Sharon.

[Child has responded, so adult moves on to the next bit of the story.]

Level 1

And we were playing on the …

Using VOCAs

Voice output communication aids (VOCAs) are extremely versatile and can be used at any point in the story. We use Big Macks (see Figure 4.2). These are the simplest and most robust aids, which record one message at a time. Because of the amount of repetition in a shared story, you can easily build in the recording of a message as you go.

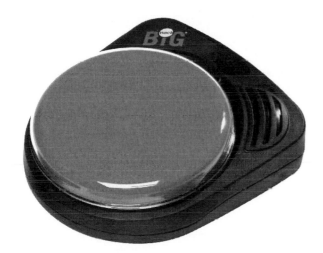

Figure 4.2 A Big Mack

We went to the (record the word 'playground' on the Big Mack). Then pass it to the child to press. If the child does not do so spontaneously, you can put the VOCA under the child's hand or against their foot or head, and move it up so that the child inadvertently activates it. We found that, after doing this for about a month, a young woman, who had no independent movement at first, started to move her fingers to activate the Big Mack herself.

There are other devices on the market that allow you to program sequences (eg: first press *hello*, second press *how are you*, third press *I'm fine*). The problem with these is that they may limit the flexibility and spontaneity of the story, and if the child presses at the wrong time, you may get the wrong sequence. As a complete technophobe, I also find them less easy to use. However, they are useful if you and other staff or family members are really competent with them. Sometimes VOCAs are programmed with only one message for one child so that you need several of them (this is often for a drama performance). I find it's much more flexible and responsive to keep re-recording messages as you need them in the story, so you don't tie up one VOCA for a limited purpose.

If you are working with children who have more advanced communication aids, just be careful that you don't program the whole story with one press. That is OK if the child is making a speech, but it is not good for promoting interactive storysharing in dialogue.

Using pictures and objects

It is really tempting to reinforce the story with lots of pictures and objects. What then happens is that the child is likely to name what she sees in the picture, or to become distracted by the objects' properties, so that you lose the intimate dynamic relationship between teller and listener. Having one or two pictures as a reference point is fine: for example, one home that we have worked with has a set of single laminated photos on a keyring, each of which stands for a story. Photos can be useful to stand for the names of people and places when children can't verbalise these. For example, you might say: 'Well, Avi was at home with [Avi shows photo] his auntie yesterday, when …'.

Using the whiteboard

The problem with technology is that it is so powerful that it can take over. Of course, the interactive whiteboard is great for getting children's attention and helping them to remember, through the pictures and videos that you show. But the same caveat applies. Once you sit children in a semicircle, looking at you and the whiteboard, you have lost the 'telling space', and this is not at all the same as sharing an experience through collective reminiscence.

Of course, you can use the whiteboard, particularly for building up the memories of what happened. But then you need to put it to one side, and tell the story together. The whiteboard needs to be inside the child's head!

Digital stories and social media

There are now a range of creative storytelling apps for tablet computers, iPads and mobile phones, and as a society we are becoming increasingly media literate. So we tell stories together by calling up images and even video sequences to incorporate as we narrate face-to-face; and we use the internet to exchange experiences with friends, family and colleagues. In Openstorytellers, we have been exploring the use of apps to help children with special needs create and tell their stories; and we are still learning!

These are powerful and attractive tools – so, just as with the whiteboard, it's important that they don't take over from the empathetic person-to-person telling. We have also found that these young people have difficulty in switching attention from device to person and back again. Remember that they have often not had the grounding in everyday person-focused telling that our media-savvy teenagers take for granted. However, we do think that apps can provide a really good and exciting, fun way of exploring and recording stories, used in conjunction with Storysharing®.

Warning: coercion

The conversational techniques we advocate have one disadvantage – it may feel somewhat coercive. Basically you are insisting that the child makes some contribution to the shared story. I don't make any apologies for this, because we are going to break down the substantial barriers caused by learned helplessness, we do need to face children with challenges and an expectation that they can and will take their rightful place in a social group. However, it is important to be sensitive, which is where the rehearsal period comes in handy. This is where you can negotiate and discuss with the child – if she wants to tell the story; who she wants to tell it to; what contribution she can and will make.

You have to take some risks and read the child's responses. If the child:

- never activates the communication aid or orientates towards it

- turns away, shuts her eyes or screams

- is persistently distracted

then you need to think again and talk with the child about how and when to tell the story, find a different story to tell, or move to one-to-one sessions.

Some children may benefit from taking part only in a very small bit of the story, or joining in from the perimeter of the group (see Chapter 5 for adapting Storysharing® to working with different groups of children).

Other techniques

There are various tricks and techniques that we have found helpful in stimulating contributions from children.

1 Deliberate forgetting

I have to say that, as I get older, this becomes increasingly natural and less contrived in my storysharing. Basically, what you do is pretend to forget a key aspect of the story that you know the child can contribute.

For example:

> *So yesterday we went to… oh gosh, where was it? It was um … tip of my tongue … umm [click your fingers] the umm, oh yeah, P…*

> *Child: Prior Park.*

(This is best with specific names of people and places, since these are the ones we habitually forget.)

2 Deliberate mistakes

You have to be careful here that the child is absolutely confident in the facts of the story, or else she is likely to agree when you get it wrong.

> *So we were in the playground at Prior Park and we went on the seesaw.*

Wait for the child to correct you; if she doesn't, revert to forget mode:

> *Oh no, hang on, it wasn't the seesaw, it was the sw …*

3 Ask for corroboration

You are allowed to ask the occasional question which will act as a prompt for the child, making sure that the last option is the correct one:

> *I think we went on the – um, was it the seesaw first or the swings? We were going to – oh gosh, where were we going? Do you remember?*

4 Rhetorical questions

Once you have got the hang of *never* asking questions, you can introduce a few of them as the conversation demands.

> *So you were on the swings, weren't you?*

> *So I was really scared, wasn't I?*

Look to the child to corroborate by nodding, smiling. These types of prompt are good at the beginning when you are working out the story, but don't rely on them, otherwise you will find you are telling the story completely and all the child is doing is nodding.

Responsive listeners

Storytellers, I always say, are like vampires. We are always hunting new blood; in this case, new listeners who have not yet heard our best stories. So with the child we go and find a listener. This might be the rest of the class, or it might be a visitor to the school, or the secretary in the office, or a friend, or the caretaker – anyone who has a bit of time to listen. You need to train your audience in the art of listening.

We are used to thinking of listening as keeping still and quiet. Good listening involves:

- eyes looking

- ears open

- mouth zipped shut

- hands on table or lap

- no fidgeting

- no talking.

Of course, this is appropriate in some class situations, but this is not actually how people behave when they are listening to an anecdote. We teach active listening, in which the only requirement is that you focus totally on the person and respond to them, rather than planning your own brilliant contribution. (Don't we all have experience of unsatisfactory audiences doing just that?)

Activity

If you have been collecting observations in your notebook, you should have some examples of active listening behaviour. List them here.

You should have noticed some or all of the following actions:

Body orientation

People shift so that they are orientated towards the telling space – that intimate triangle created between anecdotal tellers. They may lean forward and back during the telling. They tend to look at the person telling, although during a long story they may briefly look away. They will move forward and then keep still during the dramatic bits of the story.

Mirroring

When two people are telling together, and when the listeners are very involved, they often mirror the gestures and body orientation of the teller. So if the teller is using his hands to show how two cars collided, the listeners will often raise and move their own hands slightly.

Facial expressions

Listeners copy the expressions of the teller, and also react to the emotions in the story, by opening mouths, raising eyebrows, smiling and laughing, pursing lips, shaking heads.

Vocalisations

These nonverbal behaviours are accompanied by sounds such as blowing out air, tutting, and feedback responses such as *mm, hmm, uh-huh, ooh, oh*. Note that deaf signers also vocalise like this during storytelling.

Verbal feedback

Common responses include: *yeah, well, wow, no, great, really, excellent, brilliant, awesome, that's terrible/awful*.

Repetitions

Listeners repeat quite a lot of what the teller says, sometimes with a questioning intonation. *A dog? You fell over? Licked you?* For children with special needs, these repetitions are really useful as they validate what the child has said, buy her a bit of time to go on to the next bit, and serve to embed these elements of the story even more effectively. Gestures and actions are often echoed as well.

Tellers rely on these responses to keep the story going. So we need to train our audience to supply them. We have found that a few key phrases on a Big Mack are really useful – *oh no* and *wow* seem to cover most possibilities.

Listeners' reactions are not only important in keeping the story afloat, they are also barometers for ourselves about the impact of our actions.

Repeat the story

Telling the story once is not enough, as we all know. A good story demands to be repeated, with slight tweaking for new audiences. If my 18-month-old granddaughter needs to tell her duck story 30 times before she can do it on her own, how many times will it take a child with severe learning disabilities?

Your aim is to keep telling the story and gradually enable the child to take over more and more of the telling. This will happen over time because the more we tell the story, the more it becomes embedded as a script, so that we have to pay less attention to recalling the events in sequence, and can pay more attention to the audience and making the story better. So, over time, we want to shift the balance so that the shared story has minimal contributions from us and maximum ones from the child (see Figure 4.3).

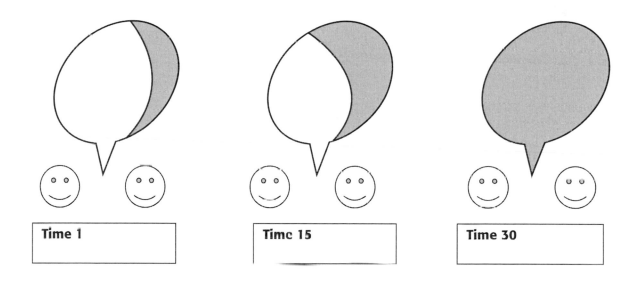

Figure 4.3 Changes in the balance of telling over time

You may also find that, over time, the child will add something to the story. For example, Adelaide's duck story at 18 months went through three stages.

Adelaide's duck story (A is Adelaide, M is mum, G is grandma)

A: Duck throw.

M: Yes, we went down to the bridge, didn't we, and we threw some ...

A: Bread.

M: Bread to the …

A: Ducks.

M: Yes, and what did you do?

A: Eat.

M: That's right, you ate the bread grandma had bought for the ducks!

A then says 'duck throw' approximately 30 times between tea and breakfast the following morning. Then she adds:

Duck throw eat.

She says this several more times, and then suddenly says:

Duck throw eat sausages.

M and G laugh.

M: You didn't eat sausages at the ducks!

G: We had sausages for tea when we came home.

A (grinning): Duck throw eat – sausages!

What had probably been an elision in the telling (Adelaide clearly knew that sausages were eaten at home rather than at the millpond) gets repeated for effect because it made us laugh.

Similarly, a man with learning disabilities who was telling a story about the bus getting stuck, which we had told and enjoyed many, many times, suddenly threw himself on the floor and announced 'Mud!' The audience, who were new to the story, responded in a most gratifying way: 'Oh no, you fell down! In the mud!'

To which I responded 'B, you so did not fall down!', and this became part of the telling of the story. This is because stories are social practices – the emphasis is as much on the impact of the telling as it is on the exact memory.

Summary

In this chapter we have:

- distinguished between the processes of finding out the facts of the story and telling the story

- identified conversational strategies to use when supporting a child to tell

- described how to rehearse and practise

- described how to tell

- identified the skills involved in being an active listener.

Activity

Go and try out these ideas. Start with an ordinary conversation. Switch between asking questions about the story, and storysharing. Note the differences.

Some examples of stories can be found in Appendix 4.

When you are confident with the techniques, try them out with some children you know.

Finally, try them out with children or adults who have communication difficulties.

Notes

9   I am grateful to a participant at the AGOSCI conference, Canberra, in May 2009 for this idea.

10 See the description under 'Using VOCAs' below.

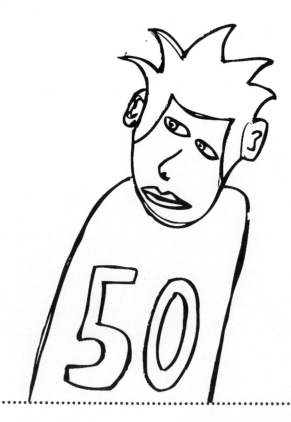

Speechmark

Storysharing®
in practice

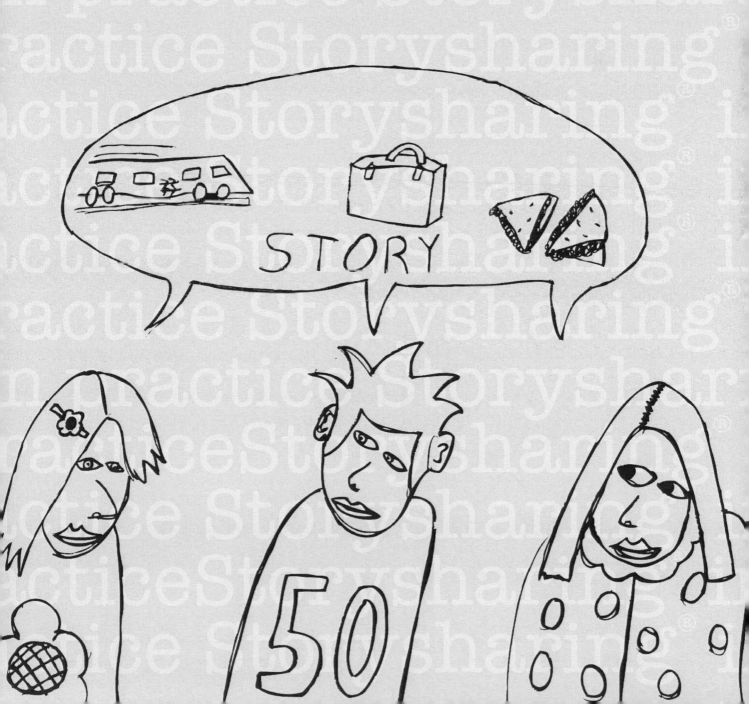

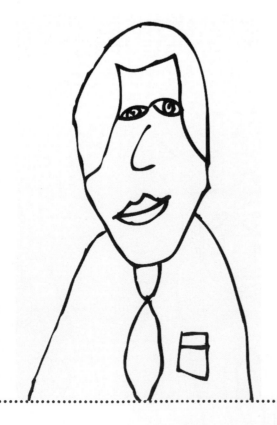

Introduction

In this chapter we look at how narrative develops in typical children and the implications for using Storysharing® with children at different levels of ability and with different special needs. We also look at how to work with individuals and with groups.

Narrative development

Preverbal development[11]

'True' narrative sequences do not begin until a child is well into her second year of development, once she can recall and produce two words in sequence. However, the roots of narrative and story can be traced back much earlier, to the expression of states and feelings (beginning as soon as the child is born) and the rhythmic exchanges that occur between infants and caregivers from about six weeks onwards, developing into quite elaborate game sequences well before the child can talk. These form the foundations on which interactive story dialogues will build, and they are as much a part of storytelling as the narratives of the events themselves.

The next significant advance for storytelling is the child's awareness of novel and unexpected happenings. This awareness emerges, of course, far earlier than narrative sequences, and first becomes actively integrated into a communicative exchange when the child draws the attention of another person to an event or object of interest, typically through pointing, reaching, laughing, looking towards the adult.

Implications for storysharing with prelinguistic children

- They will be sensitive to the *rituals* of a story: how you come together regularly and sit in a circle; how you signal that a story is beginning and ending.

- They will recognise and respond to the *feeling* elements, as conveyed through intonation, pitch changes, and associated multisensory input.

- They will gain through repeated experience of the story, and may learn to recognise the meaning of particular words and phrases.

- They may be able to participate through imitation, through gesture, through the use of voice output devices or switching to operate sound and visual effects.

- They can use objects and show pictures if you support them.

Verbal development – single words

Once children begin to use single words, they will name aspects of an event, and come quite quickly to refer to past events as well as present ones. Of course this will start with the immediate past – Hester at 14 months pointed to the liquidiser that her grandfather had just operated and went 'rrrrr' with a circular movement of her hand, then pointed to him. Children start by naming the most significant event, the high point, rather than the beginning of the story – that is, they start in the middle and have to be supported to work backwards to the start. The way that parents scaffold their children's stories at this early stage has a profound effect on subsequent narrative development and style of narrating: children of parents who focus on the emotions and the meaning of the story, or the structure of the story, tend to use these elements in their later narratives (Kelly & Bailey, 2013; Tulving & Craik, 2000).

Implications for children at single words/signs/picture or symbol use

- They will be able to use single words, and possibly short learned phrases, to describe events: first the immediate past, then, with practice, the distant past. You need to create events with them and then do immediate recall.

- They will be able to understand and use some of the language of the story.

- They will be able to direct others in a storytelling event – tell everyone to come and sit down.

- They will be able to respond to prompts and questions about the event when you are putting the story together: first *where, who, what happened*; then later *when, how* and *why*.

- They will be able to collaborate in telling their stories if you scaffold them by providing them with the lead-ins and creating a space for them to contribute.

- They will be able to show you how characters feel in a story: basic emotions such as *happy, sad, angry, proud, amused, loving*.

Verbal development – two-word stage

Once they can put two ideas together, at approximately 18 months, children begin to independently produce narrative sequences. Again, they are likely to start with the high point, and then revert back to the beginning; they may also produce 'leapfrog' narratives where they jump prematurely to the end of the story. They can respond to questions and prompts about what happened. They are more motivated to tell personal than fictional stories, and are particularly keen on negative experiences, such as accidents. (This links to other research suggesting that narratives about positive events are less structured than those about negative events: Hudson *et al*, 1992; Miller & Sperry, 1988).

Implications for children at the two to three-word level

- They will be able to provide a sequence of two- or three-word (sign/symbol) sentences that involve the key elements of a narrative, such as: Person/Object + Action (*dad run*); Action + Object (*eat cake*); Person + Place (*me school*) Action + Place (*swim seaside*); Person/Object/Place + Descriptor (*big dog*).

- They will be able to use some story conventions and stock phrases such as *Listen to me; Guess what? Once upon a time; Happy ever after.*

- They will be able to take more responsibility in narrative (one-to-one and in groups) by starting off the story and providing information about the main events. They will still need you to fill in the gaps and help them keep the story balloon in the air.

- They will be able to use *and then* to link their own sequence, with plenty of modelling and prompting: *and then, so, but.*

Later development[12]

3–4 years

Children use structural components of the story – starting with *where* and *who* and *what happened*. At first, events may not be in sequence, and information may be left out. Their narratives are often very expressive, with lots of intonation and gesture and facial expression. They begin to spontaneously link events with *and, then.*

5–6 years

Children regularly include setting statements (when and where the event happened), and begin to organise stories around the central event.

Awareness of psychological causality develops, ie that emotions give rise to actions; that certain situations cause emotions, and that actions are undertaken in pursuit of goals. Reference may be made to the intentions of characters and the future. By age 6, children can produce complete structured narratives. The range of narrative types produced by 5-year-olds in one study included *personal anecdotes; anecdotes about others, eg tattletales; routines; scripts; retellings; fantasy; pretend play narratives; deceptions and jokes* (Preece, 1987).

6–9 years

Awareness develops that people change as a result of what happens to them. Children's narratives become more complex, with awareness of the distinction between appearance and reality (deceit and trickery), multiple meanings, and the distinction between literal and figurative language. Stories become more elaborate, with multiple episodes, and represent more than one point of view. Insight into complex relationships between characters and context develops, leading to unpredictable events. Children understand the need to provide explanations for events and behaviour; and more complex emotions – jealousy, guilt; and time frames – days, weeks.

Narrative skills continue to develop in childhood, and it's obvious that adults can also develop their storytelling abilities by learning from others, such as skilled practitioners. In cultures that privilege storytelling, this is more common than in our own.

Adapting Storysharing® for different special needs

We are concentrating here on practical ways of working with three groups who can present challenges for storysharing: profound disabilities, autistic spectrum disorders, and children who use sign languages and systems. A good review of narrative issues for children with special needs can be found in Liles (1993), although the focus is largely on cognitive approaches.

Sharing stories with children who have profound and multiple disabilities

Your basic approach is to take the advice for working with prelinguistic children, but you will probably need some extra strategies to manage the additional sensory impairments, such as epilepsy, visual impairment and possibly dual sensory impairments.

Epilepsy – the child's ability to attend consistently to events will be interrupted and, of course, the drug regime will affect her concentration and motivation. There is not much you can do about this other than to take advantage of the times that you know the child will be most alert, and to use a lot of repetition.

Visual impairments – children with profound disabilities may have visual field difficulties that will affect how they look at and process information (note the best way to present it); functional visual impairments and cortical visual impairments which will affect their ability to understand what they see. They will do better with close-up small things than with looking at large things from a distance; and if brought close to a large stimulus, they will probably attend to only the part within their immediate visual field.

Hearing impairments – children will respond better to low, rhythmic, pulsing sounds than to high-pitched, quiet sounds.

Dual sensory impairments – give the children things they can feel, touch and smell, and that will vibrate. They may still be able to pick up on tones of voice and rhythmic phrasing, so don't assume they can't respond to the human voice. If you can sit behind them, put your arms around them and let them feel you talking for them: this can be very effective (they will sense the vibrations of your voice through their backs). Keep the stories very short and the listeners in very close contact. However, watch out for:

Tactile defensiveness – children may find touch, particularly sudden touch, alarming. Go very slowly and use some of the techniques suggested for autistic spectrum disorder.

Motor impairments – being in a wheelchair really affects the extent to which you can interact with the environment. If it is possible to get the child out sometimes, and on to a bean bag where you can get into closer contact, try to do so. This is appropriate when you are working individually with the child, and where you want him to pick up on the feelings and sounds of the story. Work with the physiotherapist to find which movements the child can initiate, if any, and how best to support their participation. Use switches to operate instruments and VOCAs, bearing in mind that children with severe motor impairments are likely to have most control over their heads – hold the VOCA next to their head and allow them to move gently back to contact it. Make sure the volume is not too loud as this can be distressing. Practise this with them before telling the story together.

The strengths of children with profound disabilities include a sense of humour – they will often laugh and find events funny. This suggests that your best starting point is funny stories. They benefit from exaggeration of the emotional content of the story, lots of dramatic effects, and some multisensory input (but be careful not to overdo it).

There are, of course children functioning at such an early stage, or whose responses are so compromised by their impairments, that you may feel it is tokenistic to involve them. However, do give it a try and give it time. There are two reasons for this. One is that we simply have no idea what is happening in the internal world of these children – and including them in the story of their lives is surely better than giving up. The second reason is that, although you may not see much change in the children themselves, you may find the group changes their response to them. When we included a very disabled man in a story session, we found that the others in the group started to notice him, look at him, touch him and say his name. In another case, when a man had a story to tell about going to a smart restaurant for a meal, people thought of him as the guy who had a posh meal out, as well as being the guy who makes a noise and flails around and is often difficult to calm down.

Sharing stories with children on the autistic spectrum

Usually when we tell stories we:

- centre the anecdote around an unexpected event

- aim for maximum empathy and response from our audience, so we

- emphasise the feelings

- use drama to represent what people said and did

- use a lot of gesture, facial expression and intonation

- adopt an intimate and 'resonant' body posture.

These devices are very effective for engaging the attention of children and adults with severe and profound disabilities, but for children and adults on the autistic spectrum, they are likely to prove intrusive and counterproductive. This is because they find precisely these areas difficult to handle, namely:

- unexpected events

- social responsiveness

- multichannel input.

So the strategies we have found helpful reverse all of our usual approaches.

Instead we adopt the following principles.

- Emphasise ritual.

- Emphasise the rhythmic, soothing qualities of speech, rather than use sharp changes and contrasts in intonation and pitch.

- Start with what is known.

- Use 'in repertoire' behaviours and incorporate them into the story.

- Keep the story extremely short and predictable.

- Start with routines rather than the novel event, and establish a framework for sharing a story.

- When the framework is established, introduce something new .

- In a group with other young people, allow the child with autism to join in at points and then to withdraw.

However, some of our principles still apply:

- Always talk about feelings and tell the child how you felt and how you think he felt.

- Look for positive feelings linked to experiences: love, brave, proud, exciting, funny, calm.

- Use the ritual framework to tell the story associated with negative feelings: angry, sorry, sad, scared. Always try to end with a positive.

- Repeat the story often, and repeat within the story: look for key phrases that can be used over and over again: *guess what?, oh no, oh wow, I've got something to tell you*. Put them on the Big Mack.

- Model what you want the child to do, make a space where you prompt him to join in using what you know he can do in the story.

- Emphasise how good it is to know about their experience – give them practice at telling it to others.

- Use the Big Mack.

- Use simple props.

On a training course, we discussed the following ways of involving children with severe ASD.

Ritual phrases

Matt loves … ['swimming' on Big Mack, Matt presses it.]

Joe loves … ['swimming' on Big Mack, Joe presses it.]

Sarah loves … ['swimming' on Big Mack, Sarah presses it.]

We all love … ['swimming' on Big Mack, Matt presses it.]

The teacher or other supportive adult completes the story with the novel elements, particular to each child. You start in the present (*We love swimming*) and then relate the story of a particular swimming trip, in the past. This is very important because we want to build up the children's understanding of the idea of a discrete event. We do this very slowly and it does not matter if you do the same story each time.

When Matt went ['swimming' on Big Mack, Matt presses] he jumped in. Splash. Well done Matt.

When Joe went ['swimming' on Big Mack, Joe presses] he held on tight. Well done Joe.

When Sarah went ['swimming' on Big Mack, Sarah presses] she went up and down. Well done Sarah.

Use gesture to show what the children did. Keep your voice very regular and even and slow and, over time start to introduce more intonation, so that you build in some excitement.

Over time, introduce a second Big Mack, or just rerecord, so that the children start to put in what they did as individuals.

Working with very isolated individuals

Note what they do and make it into a little story about them.

With one very autistic young man (Terry), I just sat a little distance away and said a poem – he only liked walking and he liked and knew his keyworker, Miles.

Terry went for a walk

He went up, he went down

He went round and round and round

He saw Miles

He went up, he went down

He went round and round and round

Miles and Terry came home.

Only after he had heard this about 30 times, and seemed to like it, did I introduce the Big Mack, just for his name.

Using their own behaviours

We talked about using the gesture of one young man and turning it into a story:

> *When Ravi does this [prompt him to make his usual gesture] it can mean 'go away'.*

> *When Ravi does this [prompt to make his usual downward gesture] it can mean 'sit by me'.*

Just start with this, over and over again. Make it fun; say it whenever he spontaneously makes the gesture. If he doesn't like this, say something different and much much shorter. Keep it rhythmical and verse-like. Or sing it and move gradually from song to speech. Then move into a specific event.

> *When Ravi does this [prompt him to make his usual push away gesture] it can mean 'go away'.*

> *When Ravi does this [prompt to make his usual downward gesture] it can mean 'sit by me'.*

> *Today Ravi did this [prompt the downward gesture].*

> *So I sat down with Ravi.*

> *And we just chilled!*

Working with verbal autistic children[13]

Use the same principles that we use for children with severe difficulties, but you can obviously work with their verbal skills. They may enjoy the routine, ritual and patterned aspects of the story. Estelle Keen (2004) did some research with a group of six verbal autistic children over a week, working on personal narratives which they told her on the first day. She broke down the story into episodes – day 2 beginning, day 3 middle, day 4 end, day 5 whole story told to class – and negotiated with the children to find whichever strategies they enjoyed to tell more of the story. Some children chose to draw, some to act and others liked using objects. By the end of the four 20-minute sessions, they all had improved in the amount of information they included.

Storysharing® with children who sign

If you are working with children who are reliant on sign language, you should make sure that you involve a fluent signer to help them develop good narrative skills. Narrative in sign has its own structure, which is different from that of speech. Children need to be able to manage the language space, introducing characters and organising their relationship to each other and to the locations in the story. Children with learning difficulties who use sign systems such as Makaton or Signalong (both Sign Supported English systems) will probably be using speech as well, but will benefit from using sign and gesture creatively. The same conversational strategies will help them develop their narratives.[14]

Storysharing® with children who are dependent on VOCAs

Children who have to access a communication device to give you information may also be capable of some vocalisation, eye gaze or body movement to signal how they felt or the meaning of the story. Try to encourage them to use all of their resources, even if they do this sequentially (because it requires too much effort to do both at the same time).

When working with a partner, think about giving them different roles in the story at different times – so that one child tells you what factually happened: *'Mrs Smith had gone to sleep'*, another child shows you the emotional reactions: *'Ssh!, smiling, OWWW'*, and another child shows you what they did (up-ends the watering can)[15].

Having considered ways of adapting the approach for different children, let's look at how you might implement some regular sessions, with either individuals or groups.

Working with individuals

Using the principles of intensive interaction (see www.intensiveinteraction.co.uk), provide lots of short, focused, playful sessions where you get the child used to the ritual of storysharing.

These principles include:

• Let the child take the lead.

• Imitate and echo what the child does, contingently (that is, immediately after the child's behaviour).

• Prolong your imitation of what the child is doing.

- Extend by adding in a novel element if the child is attending to you and imitating his or her in-repertoire behaviour.

- Use co-active movement (this is where you move in synchrony with the child, often with body contact) and vocalisation where you join in with the child.

- Then pause and wait for the child to notice the pause, and start again.

- Always show positive regard and respect.

Don't wait to programme a session into the curriculum – take advantage of odd moments when you and the child are together.

Working with groups

Set aside a special time

Make sure you have enough time for the group to relax into telling the stories and that there is an opportunity to share a good story with a new audience. Assemblies and parent visits are great opportunities for this. Friday afternoons, when you review what has happened in the week, are good. First thing in the morning is only good if you are prepared to spend the time – there is nothing worse than checking your watch because you have to start your project about the Vikings.

Appoint someone

Someone needs to take responsibility for running the session and putting the stories together. It may help to have a couple of people who can work together and support each other.

Group composition

Aim for a mixed ability level – the group should include children who can use a few words or signs as well as children with high support needs, because they will act as a model or catalyst for the group. A child whose behaviour can be challenging may join the group if there is appropriate support – allow them to dip in and out of the session.

Story helpers

You can bring in older children who are verbal as story helpers. Give them some basic preparation so that they know what to expect and show them how to support their friends, for example by passing an object, holding the Big Mack, joining in as listeners. In one project we gave these children certificates – and were surprised at how sensitive and insightful they were in responding to the needs of their peers.

Storysharing® for inclusion

Telling stories together offers opportunities for inclusion. We ran small groups of children with and without special needs to record and tell personal stories. Over quite short periods of time, the children learned to listen to each other, to remember each other's stories – and how to communicate successfully. Their narrative skills developed as well (Grove *et al*, 2010).

Family stories

Talk to families and carers about stories from the past – this is a wonderful link with families, who have said that they value the opportunity. It enables you to find out more about the children and gives them a history to share with others. You will, however, need to spend some time with families so that they really understand what you mean by a story. We had great success in one school with a family project where parents sent in a short story each week and we then re-enacted it in the class.

Record the stories

Have a big book or story box so that you build up a repertoire of stories. This really builds group identity. And then:

Tell them over and over again!

Troubleshooting

Working with personal stories is highly creative and rewarding – but not without its challenges! Here are a few problems we have come across, with some ideas for tackling them.

What happens if ...

Children don't respond

Remember, it takes time for people to become familiar with a new challenge and to learn what is expected of them.[16] It's the same with intensive interaction. Trust the process, even if it takes some time. Storysharing® is a social process. If you value the session, so will they. If you find it boring or unproductive, so will they.

I feel silly clowning around when children don't seem to notice

All work with children with high support needs involves some risk-taking on our part if it is going to be anything other than routine and predictable. Again, think of this as a kind of Intensive Interaction (Nind & Hewett, 2005). Notice and comment on what the child did at the time of the event. What you are trying to do is to help them remember, at some level and in some way, an experience. It's one of the most important things you can do for and with them. If you can enjoy the session, they will too.

The only event involves bad behaviour that we don't want to reinforce

This is a very common problem – and an obvious strategy is to make sure that there are some alternative, positive events in the child's life that can be shared. It may be possible to use the peer group to express sanctions – this, after all, is the most effective way of changing behaviour. That is, the child tells the story, perhaps to a couple of older, more able story helpers, who respond appropriately. Typically developing children would be engaged in this sort of interaction all the time. Sharing the difficult things we do as well as the good things may be possible if you can set up a really supportive, confidential group – using a circle of friends or circle time principles (see the websites www.inclusive-solutions.com/circlesoffriends.asp; www.circle-time.co.uk).

The event was distressing or sad – I'm not sure I should be revisiting it

This is a tricky one. We should, however, be wary of thinking that because we never refer to what happened, the child is not affected in some way by it. It may be healthier to accept that some events do make us sad or upset – and treat it in a low-key way, by reflecting the feelings back – *This is what happened. It made you sad. It makes me sad too. It's OK to feel sad.*

You can stay with sad or upsetting feelings, using colour (eg a black velvet cloth), quiet music, or an object associated with the sad event. A similar approach can be used for anger (a red cloth, spiky texture, helping them to drum or use a cymbal). You might want to liaise with drama, play or music therapists to work through some of these events, or enable the child to work with a counsellor.[7] Follow this retelling with something you know the child likes – nice food, a cup of tea, dancing to music.

The child has got stuck on the same story

The desire to tell and retell the same story in exactly the same way is very common. Sometimes this is because it is just the favourite story, but sometimes the perseveration reflects an underlying obsession, anxiety or preoccupation. The child may resist any modifications. You need to look for ways of either building in some tiny changes, which gradually provide an alternative story path, or a way of developing the story.[8] For example, with one person who kept talking about his fears of staff cuts, we took his worries seriously and wrote a letter to the MP, which resulted in the whole group having a tour of the House of Commons. This meant that when he started on his story, we could take it a bit further – 'Yes, and you wrote to … MP, we put the letter in the … [postbox], etc'. You may be able to add codas to a story – along the lines of what someone would like to happen to change things, or hopes to do. Bear in mind that once a story has been told, it does in a sense belong to the listener too – so you can legitimately chip in with your own responses and reactions as you tell collaboratively: When Jenny says, repeatedly, 'I watch Dr Who. Hide behind the sofa. I'm scared of the Daleks', you may be able to add in:

> Dr Who is scary. After 'Dr Who' it was 'Weakest Link'. Jenny said "Goodbye!"

or:

> Usually Jenny watches [Dr Who] but when it's not on, she …

or:

> I'm scared of Daleks too so I don't watch it, I watched …

If the story relates to something that routinely happens in the week, which just gets rehearsed, try to build in a very small change to the routine and incorporate it in the story. If you think there is a real underlying issue for the child, you may want to involve a play therapist.

The child does not seem to know the difference between fantasy and reality

Imagination plays a large part in children's stories and, once you open the door to the freedom of telling, a child may well introduce fantasy elements and blur the boundaries. This is part of typical development (Engel, 1995; Fox, 1993) and, of course, much great children's literature is based on precisely this premise. The imaginative development of the story may not reflect what happened in the physical world, but it will be firmly rooted in the child's emotional reality. We also need to be aware that selective interpretation and elaboration of the factual truth is characteristic of anecdotal narratives. Of course, we tend to blur the distinction ourselves because we will say 'That's a great story' for both imaginative fictions and anecdotes of real experience. You can help by the way you reinforce what the child says: 'Yes, that really happened!', 'That didn't really happen, but what an exciting thing to think of'. The social context is critical – making sure that there is a place where children can make up stories and transform reality, which is clearly demarcated, both as a physical and a social space, from the space where you tell personal anecdotes. The collaborative approach also helps to ground the child, because you are remembering together and checking each other's memories. You can also use rehearsal time to draw distinctions – 'Let's tell what really happened first, and then what you thought might happen'. And again, bear in mind that some children may need more dedicated input from play or drama specialists or therapists.

Nothing happened this week

Well, there is always something that happens, however trivial. You can make a drama out of the tiniest thing, and often this is a way of getting people involved in their own lives. For example, you mislay the keys to the van – find a child, tell them about it, get them to look for the keys somewhere. Yes, this takes time – but actually they might enjoy a dramatic search for keys which they eventually produce with a flourish, just as much as the actual trip in the van. If you haven't got a story on the morning of the session – create one!

For example: Drop something on the floor; spray yourself with tap water and get soaking wet, and get everyone to dry you off; bang your head on something and get everyone to rub it better; put on two different shoes; wear a red nose; get locked out, and shout at the window until a child notices; wrap up a parcel of goodies and discover it on the doorstep; refuse to do any cleaning and get all the children to gang up on you to shout with a Big Mack 'Don't be lazy'; get someone to park their car in an annoying place so that wheelchairs can't get out of the front door, take the children out and have them push against the car, then shout for the owner using a Big Mack; go out shopping and forget your list, having given everyone you are taking a picture of what is needed beforehand so that they can remind you.

The children are inventing things that aren't true

As we have noted, children may elaborate or add things to a story that did not actually happen. Staff tend to get very worried about the boundaries between fantasy and reality, because obviously some children find it difficult to do this. However, remember the following.

Sharing personal stories is a social practice

This means that the act of telling is as important as the memory itself – and is somewhat different from the memory. In fact, over time, as we tell our favourite anecdotes, they float off from the real events and assume a life of their own through the telling. We all embroider a good story and tinker around the edges. What this means is that you can tolerate a degree of exaggeration if the central core of the story remains true. You can also build your own corrections into the telling of the story, as I did with the man who added 'falling down in the mud'.

Summary

In this chapter we have:

- seen how narrative develops in childhood

- considered the implications of this information for Storysharing® with children at different stages of development

- identified some issues and strategies for working with children who have profound and multiple disabilities and children with autism

- considered how to tell stories with individuals

- considered how to tell stories in groups.

Notes

11 For preverbal and early development of narrative, see Bates, 1976; Ellis, 2007; Miller & Sperry, 1988; Scollon, 1979; Weir, 1962.

12 Summaries of later narrative development can be found in Liles, 1993; Preece, 1987; Nippold, 2007; for overviews of narrative development, see the relevant chapters in Bamberg, 1997; Engel, 1995; McCabe & Bliss, 2003; Peterson & McCabe, 1983.

13 I am indebted to Peter & Sherratt Smith, 2001 for the general principles of using creative and imaginative ideas with children on the autistic spectrum.

14 For sign language development, see Schick et al, 2006; for the assessment of narrative skills in signers, see Herman et al, 2004; for narratives in sign by children with intellectual disabilities, see Grove & Tucker, 2003.

15 The idea of role separation came from a workshop at Corseford school in Glasgow (so did the story!) and discussions with Annalu Waller and Rolf Black, University of Dundee.

16 In my experience, it can sometimes take three or four sessions for children to process what is going on and then respond. This is a bit like listening to a new piece of music – the first time you hear it, you don't think it is anything much to write home about; by the third time, you are beginning to hum the tune.

17 In rare cases, the child may disclose information that you feel should be passed to another authority; your school or organisation must have procedures for dealing with such a situation.

18 Peter & Sherratt Smith (2001) give some guidelines about how to help children develop their stories and imaginative play.

CHAPTER 6

Assessing progress and planning intervention

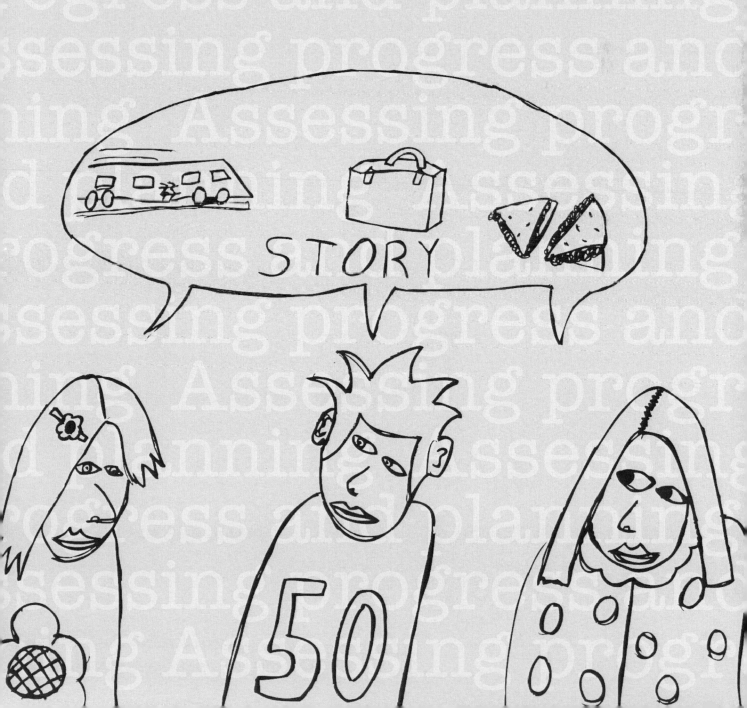

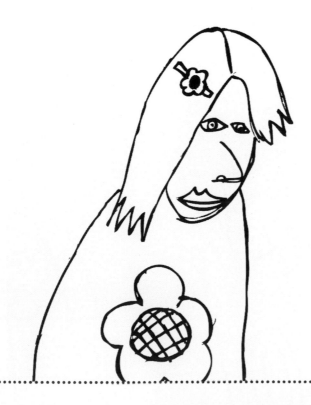

Introduction

This chapter presents a framework for assessing children's skills in sharing stories over time and considers how to plan interventions based on the assessment.

About assessment

There are different ways of assessing children's skills, depending on why you are carrying out the assessment. For example, you might want to find out if the child has a problem or is particularly good at telling stories. Standardised tests, which are reliable to administer and give you a score, are one way of doing this. The score will tell you how the child compares with other children of the same chronological or mental age. These sorts of tests are 'standardised'; that is, the table of scores is based on the test having been administered in exactly the same way to large groups of children of different ages. This means there are very strict rules about how the test should be carried out. Usually, the test involves the children making up a story from wordless pictures, or remembering a story you have told them. These results don't always relate very closely to what the children can do with personal stories in informal situations when they are motivated and excited to share their experiences.

In Storysharing® we don't use this kind of test. Instead, we encourage the child to tell a story, with or without help. We film them, and then do very careful profiling using a framework based on the social model of storytelling. This is very flexible, and by repeating it over time (or in different contexts), you can see what progress the child is making. It will also help you to plan your intervention or teaching.

In designing our profile we have to think about:

- the tasks we are going to use to assess the child's skills and the best way of getting the child to tell the story

- the elements of narrative that we think it is important to describe – what we are going to assess.

How to get the child to tell a story

We want to know how well the child can convey a personal story. This means that we want some standard of comparison. In our assessments, we compare a negative and a positive story with the way the child narrates routines.

We expect that a routine will be:

- a sequence of events

- told using the present tense

- told with relatively little emotion.

This is the easiest kind of narrative to elicit.

With personal narratives, ask the child to tell you or someone else about a recent event where you know the basic outline. Start with a negative event so that you end with a positive.

Provide a story model. Tell the child briefly about something that happened to you, and then ask if anything similar has ever happened to them. Good stimuli are: going to hospital, going on holiday, getting a present, doing something naughty, or doing something really helpful.

For children who cannot do this, try a collaborative story. Find out about an event that is important to the child, and tell it with them to a new person. Rehearse it with the child first and then, during the telling, gradually reduce your level of input. Again, you can do this collaboratively if necessary.

Prompting strategies during assessment

Intervene as little as possible, but keep the child going by:

- repeating what they have said with a questioning intonation

- using non-specific prompts – *and then?*

- giving feedback responses – *mmm, oh, right, wow, yes?*

Assess both story generation and retelling

Story generation is where the child makes up a story; story retelling is where the child retells a story he has heard. You can compare the two and see whether there is a difference. Story generation would be when you ask the child to tell you his own experience. Retelling would be when you tell a personal story and then ask the child to tell it to someone else.

Appendix 3 provides an assessment protocol.

What to assess

Our framework, as discussed in Chapter 2, is based on the understanding that narrative is a socially constructed process – that is, it happens between people in a very interactive way. This model emphasises not only the very familiar structural elements of story but also the ways in which the teller conveys to the listener how they ought to be feeling and judging the events in the story.

Aspects of storytelling

Social (audience awareness)

The ability to engage and sustain the attention of an audience.

Feelings and perspectives

The ability to convey the feelings associated with the events, and to signal how the event should be viewed and judged.

Story structure

The organisation of key story elements: who, what, where, when, how, why of story.

Organisation

The recall and sequencing of events.

Language

Language that enables children to convey the story structure and feelings (verbs, adjectives, nouns, pronouns, conjunctions, clause structure).

Patterning and poetry

The conventions and rhetorical devices associated with the culture of story and audience awareness (stock phrases for opening and closing stories, metaphor). Also prosody, rhythm and intonation, and repetition for effect.

If the story is told with another person, we are also going to look at how actively they contribute, and whether their contribution changes over time or in different situations

Finally, we are going to assess their skills as *listeners* as well as tellers.

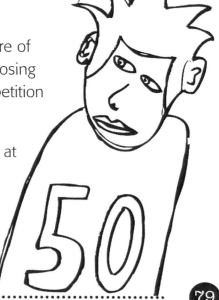

Listening

The following framework is based, for the first six levels, on Erica Brown's (1996) model of participation, and on Norrick's (2000) analysis of conversational anecdotes for levels 7–10.

The profile is provided in Appendix 5.

Framework for developing listening skills

1   *Encounter*. Being prepared to sit and attend as a member of an audience, for increasing periods of time.

2   *Supported participation.* Tolerating physical prompts for responses, eg the use of switch or musical instrument.[19]

3   *Awareness*. Noticing the storyteller or some aspect of the story such as a prop, eg making eye contact, orientating the body towards the telling space.

4   *Response*. Showing some kind of spontaneous response to some aspect of the story or the teller, eg laughing, imitating sound or movement.

5   *Engagement*. Directed attention, focused looking, listening, showing interest, recognition or recall.

6   *Involvement*. Active participation – reaching out, joining in with the story.

7   *Feedback*. Giving back channel responses: nodding, co-active gestures, leaning forwards, saying 'oh no, really?, wow!' at appropriate points.

8   *Exploration*. Questioning and commenting: monitor the storyteller and ask for clarification and elaboration of key points.

9   *Co-narration.* Taking up an opportunity to contribute to the story, eg show us how you put out your hand for the bus; say what you said to your mum.

10 *Response story*. Tell all or part of a story which is related to some element of a preceding narrative.

Levels 7–10 require the listener to follow the story and attend over time to the content, as well as to the teller. These represent very big steps pragmatically for individuals with communication difficulties. Nevertheless, the skills involved can be prompted at first, and scaffolded by a story helper.

This profile is provided in Appendix 5.

Recording

Use video if you can, because you will want to look at gesture and facial expressions as well as what the child says. The record form can be used to profile the child's strengths and needs as a storyteller, and to identify particular targets.

Identifying strengths and needs

Once you have a profile of the child's skills in each area, you can identify their relative strengths and needs. Use the framework to decide what you will target for intervention.

Intervention

Remember – narrative is different from 'argumentation, description and exposition'. You have to create the condition of narrative expectancy. Too many questions and prompts will disrupt the flow of the story. Learn to wait and support, rather than take over. And narrative involves *reportable* events – it must be worth the effort involved in recalling, organising the information and retelling.

Good narrators are made not born – narrative is the product of particular cultural experiences. Children need models of storytelling.

Developing the different aspects involved in telling a story

Focus on social: audience awareness and experience

Provide experiences of telling and listening, with attentive and sensitive prompting.

Help the child to take over more responsibility for telling the story. Use a collaborative approach – identify where and how the child can join in with a story; provide props to help tell it.

Focus on story structure and organisation

Help the child to organise the structure of the story, with associated work on the key elements of structure: who, where, when, what happened, how did you feel, what was said. Cue cards can be useful, with different colours to emphasise the different story elements.

Focus on feelings

Emphasise different feelings yourself as you tell the story. Name the feelings. Practise nonverbal behaviours associated with different feelings. Try saying phrases from the story in ways that convey different feelings. Play games to change voices and facial expressions.

Focus on language

Have a stock set of phrases that you use to introduce the story and at different points in stories. They can be programmed on voice output aids, which are pressed at the appropriate time and everyone can join in. The children can act as monitors to tell the audience when to come out with a particular phrase. For example:

Guess what?

Oh no!

And then …

*It was **so** awful/brilliant/funny/cool.*

On and on and on.

The language associated with story structure can be developed through the formal teaching of vocabulary such as verbs, adjectives, and sentence structure.

Focus on patterning and poetry

Sing and chant different parts of the story, emphasising the rhythm.

Play with telling the story loudly, softly, slowly, or fast.

Put conventional phrases and story language on a Big Mack.

Exaggerate intonation and prosodic contours and help the child to join in.

Encourage lots of vocalisation and rhythmic movement to go with the story.

Most of all – enjoy the story. Have fun, put your heart and soul into it, and let the children know it really matters to you to hear what they have to tell you!

Summary

In this chapter we have:

- looked at the type of assessment that is appropriate for storysharing

- considered the tasks through which we can assess the children's skills

- identified the aspects of storytelling to assess

- presented a profile

- considered intervention strategies for different types of skills.

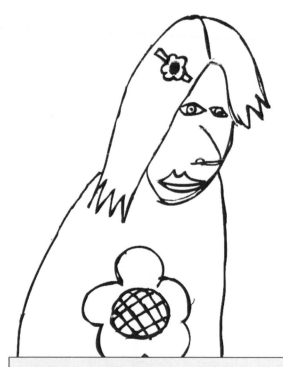

Note

19 I put this much earlier than Brown, since my experience is that this behaviour can be facilitated well before the development of spontaneous awareness or response.

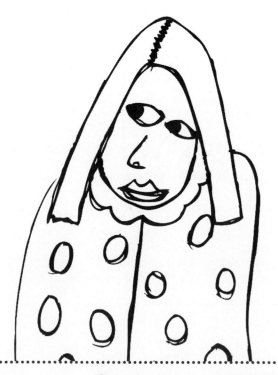

Speechmark

CHAPTER 7

Developing Storysharing®

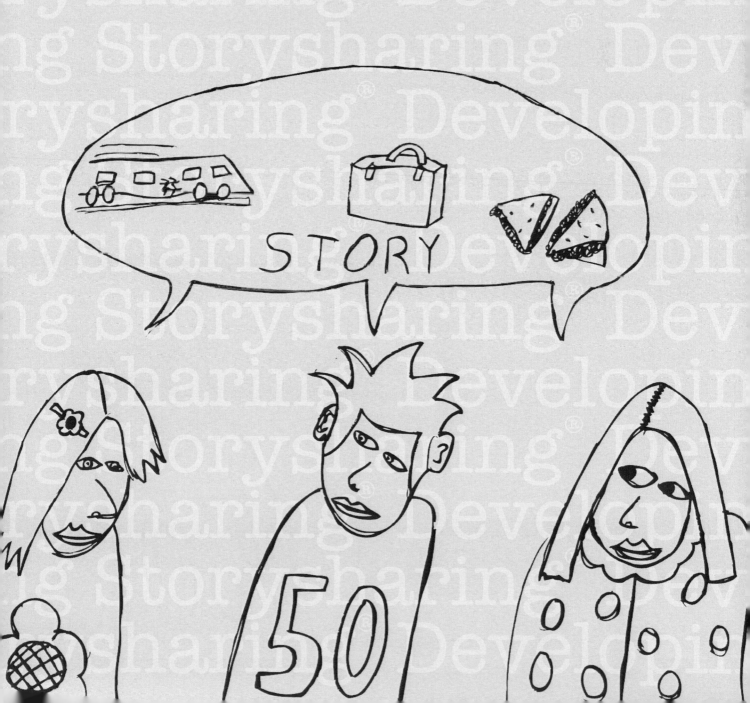

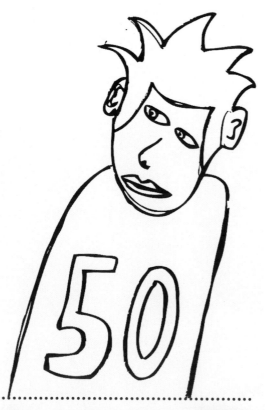

Introduction

This chapter deals with how to create an environment – at home and in school – that promotes the sharing of personal experience; and how to develop children's narratives into writing and drama – whether for the enjoyment of family and the creation of family memories, or for learning. Finally, we will identify some criteria that can be used to audit the environment: this is, of course, principally for schools and residential homes.

At home

Home is the place where stories start and finish. It's the most important place for stories to happen and be shared. Family narratives act as memory scrapbooks where the identity of the family and the people in the family is built up and developed. As families tell stories together, different views are shared, and sometimes there are arguments: see the family narrative at the beginning of this book. (For more on family narrative, see Fiese, 1999; Pratt & Fiese, 2004.)

For the families of children with special needs, there are lots of difficulties to deal with every day, and it can be hard to make the space and find the energy to tell stories. But it is really important that the children get the opportunities, to have their own stories and to share in the stories that everyone else is telling.

Activity

When do families share stories about their lives?

- When are the best times for telling stories?

- What are the times to avoid?

You have probably come up with a list that includes meals, watching the television, car journeys, visits from relatives and friends, when washing up, bathtimes, bedtimes and on the phone. And for the worst times: getting ready to go out, getting up in the morning, and during homework or computer sessions. Children won't want to tell family stories if they are going out, watching television or playing computer games, or hanging out with their friends.

The message is to use the times that occur naturally in your family to share stories together, and not to put pressure on yourselves. The best way of involving the child in stories is when you are all doing it together, and you create a space where the child really wants to contribute.

In a project I carried out a few years ago,[20] a family really got into the routine with their child of recording key events in a scrapbook to tell me about, and they would go through it in the evenings so the child could practise. Having me as a listener who really wanted to hear the news helped provide the motivation for her telling, and she loved collecting remnants to put in a 'secret' envelope – I had to guess what was in there, and what had happened.

Between home and school

The need to inform other people about what is happening in the different compartments of our lives is a powerful reason for developing narrative skills. As teachers and parents know, however, the gap can be really difficult to bridge.

Reluctant tellers

We are all familiar with the situation when the child comes home from school and, when asked what happened, says 'Nothing'. This starts really early – my 3-year-old granddaughter would give this reply when she returned from nursery, which astonished me. The last time the 5-year-old said it, it transpired that they had actually been handling snakes, which was definitely not routine in the curriculum. The answer to the reluctant teller lies (we think) in our model of storysharing – that is, rather than putting the child on the spot, or asking too many direct questions, create the conditions where the child wants to tell you something and encourage them by modelling, talking about your own day, and perhaps making some inferences from what is in their school bag.

The home–school book

Most schools have a system in which they communicate about important issues for the child by writing in a book which goes between the two settings. Usually (for very good reasons of time) these are extremely brief factual accounts. In one project, we started a system of sending back a story diary, just once a week, in which parents and teachers used the record form to give the basic information about a story that the child could tell – not a long narrative account, but just enough to enable the appropriate support to be put in place. For other children, sending a simple voice output button, or a talking photo album, is a useful alternative (see Appendix 2 for some different ways of recording stories).

At school

In a child's life at school it is the social experiences that are of primary importance – the playground, the lunch table, the seating arrangements in class and on the coach for trips out. Children who are confident narrators and listeners will have a real advantage when it comes to making and keeping friends. The structure of social spaces is of recognised importance – cosy places where children can feel secure and exchange confidences, benches to sit on, designated areas for games that involve language and negotiation (skipping rhymes and other playground scripts not only contain powerful, often transgressive, narratives but also reinforce the rhythmic patterning that we find in storytelling). In class, there are the framing sessions at the beginning and end of the day (news time, round up time), circle times, and points within particular lessons where personal anecdotes may be relevant. We'll look first at formal contexts in which narratives can be shared, and then at some of the directions that narrative might go – into drama, writing and film.

News time

The problem with news time, or 'show and tell', is that it often becomes an institutionalised start to the day. The teacher's agenda is to complete the newsround in a designated period of time, with news being delivered that is maximally relevant and maximally succinct. The child's agenda is usually to hold the floor as long as possible (alternatively, to sink out of the spotlight). Listening is not really privileged, turn-taking is – in other words, the focus is on the child's turn to talk. It should be obvious by now that news time is not necessarily (perhaps not even optimally) story time. We are inclined to reward children's contributions by saying 'What a good story', regardless of the interest level. Avoid this! Instead, make a clear distinction between news telling – the most interesting thing, told very briefly – and storysharing. For example, you might write up or draw one thing for each piece of news, and then decide which items should be told as a story, perhaps at round-up time – after a little practice with a support person. Of course, there is always news that has to be told in a more extended way, because of its significance to the child or the group.

Round-up time and assemblies

This can be at the end of the day, when the key events of the day are remembered together, using the techniques of Storysharing® – the best thing that happened, the funniest, the worst, or the best story from this morning's news. At the end of the week, you can do a reprise. Good stories can be taken to assemblies, which are the formal arena for the building of a community history and identity.

Seize the moment

Be aware during the day of any really exciting event that should be processed, recalled and storied immediately. It really is worth giving up on a maths lesson for a short period of time to take advantage of spontaneous events. We all know these – it starts to snow; someone emails a photo of the new baby; a dog wanders into the classroom; a rubbish-collection truck up-ends its load outside your window. Grab these moments – take a photo if you like but, above all, help the children to make them into stories.

Story space

Vivien Paley is a teacher who has made powerful use of story space within the classroom where children can develop their sense of themselves as narrators (Paley, 1991). This is a space where there are comfortable cushions, a table, props and drawing and writing materials, where children can go to develop their stories. Within our framework, it would act as a Storysharing space where children could work with a partner to develop their storytelling.

Curriculum

The extent to which personal narratives are included in the curriculum as a specific lesson focus varies. In the English national curriculum there has been a very overt focus on cognitive analytical skills; some would say at the expense of creative, affective and social skills. Moreover, almost everything to do with story has been located within literacy, with very little awareness of the importance of narrative talk. This imbalance has been redressed to an extent by the recognition that speaking and listening are essential as the foundation of learning and socialisation.[21] There is still an argument to be made about the importance of personal storytelling in children's lives – and we hope that this book has provided enough ammunition for you!

How Storysharing® relates to other forms of narrative

Storysharing® and sensory stories

Sensory stories has become a kind of shorthand for approaches that involve the use of props which can be touched, moved, felt, smelt or tasted, and dynamic movements, which illustrate the story and make it possible for the child to access the meaning at some level. Of course, you can use the Storysharing® approach as you are telling sensory stories. Although they were developed initially with fictional stories (children's literature and traditional legends), sensory props are increasingly used to tell children's own stories. Usually, the approach involves essentially 'reading' the story either with or to the child, with some participation. The difference between this and Storysharing® is that our emphasis is on direct, dynamic, oral telling, with props kept to a minimum. As you involve more props and more scripting, the story moves to a more structured, formalised record of what happened. This is brilliant as a way of capturing important memories.

For example, Jamie and Karen had only one really significant event in their lives: a trip to Lourdes in France. This was such an important story that we felt we should do more than just tell it together. We asked Bag Books (www.bagbooks.org.uk) to come and help us, and they created a Bag Book story, with a page and a prop to represent going on the plane, meeting the priest, going down into the dark cave, hearing the music and feeling the holy water.

In Storysharing®, the difference is that the stories are often shorter, and told with more collaboration between everyone, with more of a focus on the social aspect than on the sensory experience. Of course, as I hope you can see, both are important.

Storysharing® and drama

There is a very subtle difference between telling a story and acting a story, which can be hard to define in real life, not least because we often move into dramatisation during an anecdote – for example, miming to show how someone moved, or using dialogue. In brief, in drama, events are played out as if they were happening in front of the eyes of the audience, and the teller has to adopt different distinct roles. There are no linking units – the spectator infers the passage of time, and the connection between events. By contrast, when a story is narrated, the teller is locating the event in the past (even if the present tense is used) and framing the story for the listener. The difference is experienced as partly to do with pace and immediacy – when you dramatise the events, it feels very punchy and fast, with one event succeeding another. Storytelling is more leisurely, with an internal structure and rhythm, and the meaning is made explicit. We need both modes of narrative, of course. However, Storysharing® should not be confused with acting the story. It's better to decide between yourselves that this would make a great story to act as a play, and then assign roles. Paley uses this technique in her storytelling classrooms, and it proved very effective in a class in an SLD school.

Basically, we got in stories from families, we told them together, and then we acted them, with the focus child deciding who should play which role. For example, Mary's story was that her mum had put her dad's hammer in the fridge by mistake (yes, dear reader, you too will do this at some point in your life). Mary played herself, and other children took the role of her mum and dad. Nadia's story was about how her mum came to school when she had to have an injection. Here Nadia took the role of the nurse, with me playing her. This was really therapeutic for Nadia, who is scared of needles.

Storysharing® and literacy

We have already commented on the difference between written stories and orally told stories. What seems to happen as the stories are written down is that a lot of the elements which are distinctive to oral narrative are edited out. They may disappear altogether – for example, hesitations, false starts and repetitions. Or they may be replaced by words, as tends to happen with gestures, facial expressions and prosody. As a story is transformed into written narrative, it becomes a more organised, structured, tidier creature. Look at the following example.

Giuliana's story told (capital letters indicate marked emphasis; signs indicate British Sign Language; gesture means emphatic or spatial indication)

Giuliana (gaining attention): When I was five, when I was five, I went (signs GO) I walked to the big (gestures) big market and there were shops EVERYWHERE (gestures) and I ran (signs RUN) I ran to the toy shop, cos I liked toys, I really really liked toys to play with them (gesture) and my brother, my brother, he saw (signs) me run (signs) and he didn't say (signs NO SAY) anything to my mum and then, my mum, she said to my brother (signs CHILD), she said as a joke, she didn't really mean it (gesture), she said it as a joke (gesture) she said as a joke to my brother, she said 'Let's leave Giuliana aside (gestures) let's go home without her'. My brother – he started crying (signs CRY) he was very upset, he started crying. He RAN (signs) after me, he GRABBED me (gesture) and took me to my mum (gesture) and then my mum (wags finger) and she told me off, because I ran off (signs) without telling her. And I got told off (wags finger, shrugs).

Activity

Rewrite the example above so that it could be read as a literate story. I have had a go at the end of the chapter.

We are used to thinking of this as an advance, but for conversational anecdotes, it is a poor substitute. What gets edited out here are all the devices which are actually keeping the attention of Sally, the child with special needs with whom Giuliana is sharing the story. The repetitions, which look irrelevant on paper, are delivered with slightly differing intonation and stress changes, and they signal the high point of the story. Sally is riveted. You also miss (because I couldn't write everything down!) all of the small gestures and interactions between the two of them: Sally's reactions, the way Giuliana picks up some of the gestures that Sally had used in the immediately preceding story, which involved her getting a telling off.[22]

In fact, writers spend years and years trying to recapture authentic dialogue. It is often entirely appropriate to move from oral narrative to creative writing – but it is not always necessary. For the short, ephemeral, tiny stories of everyday life, they can be kept fresh and spontaneous by not consigning them to the page. Other stories, though, that are important to the child or the community, can be moved into a graphic form. This means writing or drawing, using pictures, apps and animated graphics, PowerPoint presentations, as well as books, diaries and screens on a VOCA. Writing does, of course, help to support the development of narrative structure.

The message is really that stories need to be told in many different ways in different contexts. We like to read and write stories, when we are the only listeners and tellers. We like to watch stories acted out, as private or public performances. And we also like to sit with our friends and say 'Remember when ...?', 'Tell the one about ...', where we actively share our reminiscences in dialogue.

The storytelling environment

What would an environment that is really conducive to storytelling look like?

Essentially, what we are trying to develop for our children is the possibility of being part of a narrative culture. So how would we recognise it when we see it?

Activity

List 10 features that you would look for in order to tell whether a classroom or home is a place where stories are told and valued.

I define a narrative culture as one where telling and listening to stories is embedded in both formal and informal practices. In a school, that would mean both in lessons and gatherings and in the playground, the dining hall, the time waiting for the bus to arrive for a trip, the staff room, the photocopier room and the tuck shop. In a home, it would involve meetings, discussions, the child's quiet private space with a trusted friend, the dining room, the kitchen, the car, where housework, shopping and gardening are being done; where the television and computer are ignored (sometimes!) in favour of animated chat. A narrative culture is where the stories that are told in the staff room are also shared with the children, and where the stories that the children tell each other are given prominence and value. Here's my list of things to look for.

1 Stories and storytelling are regarded as central to the life of the community. A range of different types of story can be observed, in different settings.

2 Reportable events are foregrounded. When something happens which represents a significant departure from routine, people take the opportunity to turn it into a story, with a beginning, middle and end and a high point.

3 Everyone is involved. There is a continuum of supported participation, so that every child has an opportunity regularly to tell a story and listen to stories, both as part of a group and one-to-one.

4 Staff tell stories to each other, children tell stories to each other, and staff tell stories with children.

5 Stories are visible. For example, there are displays relating to events and stories that have been shared in the community, presented with a narrative perspective – eg sequenced, speech bubbles, feelings mentioned. Stories are recorded in ways that are accessible to the children.

6 Children are enabled to share difficult as well as positive experiences when it is appropriate to do so. Their feelings are recognised and respected.

7 Learning is recognised. In schools or other organisational settings, there is some system for monitoring and assessing progress in the telling of stories.

8 Adults and older children know how to support younger children or children with special needs to join in a story.

9 Listeners are responsive when stories are told.

10 Stories are revisited time and time again, to develop a sense of community and identity.

You can keep track of the way in which a narrative culture is developing through carrying out a review or an audit.

Table 7.1 overleaf is a suggested template for keeping track of what personal and community stories are told. The list includes some types of story that we have found to recur in the places where we have worked – please feel free to add to it.

Review: what stories are being told now.

Plan: how you will systematically ensure that, across the school year, children are exposed to a range of different types of stories and ways of telling.

Record: the use of stories after they have happened.

The template can be used for the school as a whole, for individual children, or for individual staff members to track what they are doing or would like to do. The 'How' and 'Response' columns are included for individuals.

Where and when: the context in which this type of story could best be shared.

Who with – eg staff member, friend, family, small group, one-to-one, whole class, assembly.

How – the strategy that would best be suited to this type of story or this individual child.

Response – what you would look for in the child, how and where they might join in.

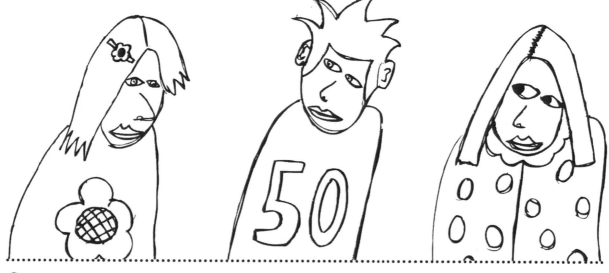

Table 7.1 Template for recording personal stories

Type of personal story	Where and when	Who with	How	Response
Holidays				
Celebrations and festivals				
Achievements				
Surprises				
Comic events				
Romantic/friendship events				
Being brave				
Illness				
Accidents				
Loss (of items)				
Getting lost or left behind				
Bereavement				
Scary events				
Frustrations				
Disappointments				
Shocks				
Rows and quarrels				
Weather				
Transport				
Food and cooking				
Shopping				
Pets				
Sibling sayings and doings				
News, ie national and local				
Dreams and fantasies				

Summary

In this chapter we have:

- considered how stories are told at home and in school

- explored the relationship between oral storytelling and drama

- explored the relationship between oral and written stories

- considered how to recognise and develop a narrative culture.

Happy storysharing!

Giuliana's story written version:

This is a story about when I was five. I used to love toys and toyshops. Well, one day I went to the market with my mum and my older brother. There were shops everywhere and they were really big. When we got there, my mum wasn't looking, and I ran off to the toyshop. My brother saw me but he didn't tell mum. Then my mum said, just as a joke, 'Let's leave Giuliana here and go home without her'. She didn't mean it. And my brother started crying and he ran to get me, grabbed me, and brought me back to mum. And she was very cross with me and told me off.

Notes

20 Family Album, 2001–2002. Funded by the Health Foundation: thanks Catherine, David and Jenny.

21 See, for example, *Speaking, Listening, Learning: working with children who have special educational needs*, which has a strong focus on narrative, at the website http://dera.ioe.ac.uk/6912/1/pns_sen118705sll.pdf

22 Example from the Storytree project which brought children from mainstream and special schools together, funded by SENJIT, the London Borough of Harrow, and Somerset Community Foundation.

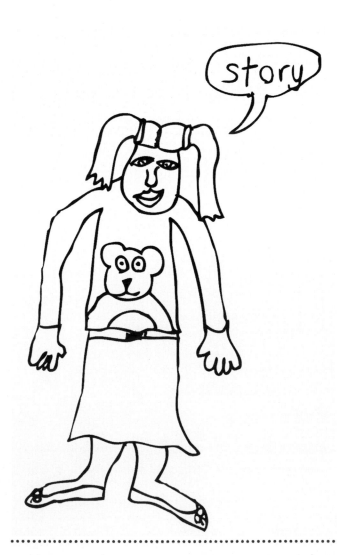

REFERENCES

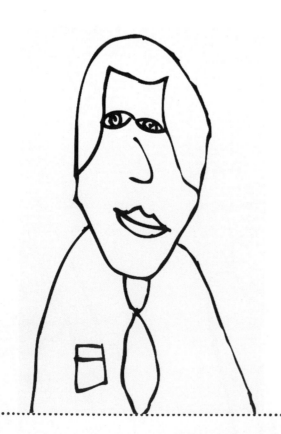

Baddeley A (1997) *Human Memory: Theory and Practice*, Psychology Press, Hove.

Bamberg M (ed) (1997) *Narrative Development: Six Approaches*, Lawrence Erlbaum Associates, Mahwah, NJ.

Bates E (1976) *Language and Context: The Acquisition of Pragmatics*, Academic Press, New York.

Booker C (2004) *The Seven Basic Plots: Why We Tell Stories*, Continuum, London.

Brown E (1996) *RE For All*, Fulton, London.

Dickinson C (1991) 'Teaching agenda and setting: constraints on conversation in preschools', McCabe A & Peterson C (eds), *Developing Narrative Structure*, Lawrence Erlbaum Associates, Hillsdale, NJ, pp255–303.

Dunbar R (1998) *Grooming, Gossip and the Evolution of Language*. Havard University Press, Havard.

Ellis L (2007) 'The narrative matrix and wordless narrations: a research note', *Augmentative and Alternative Communication*, 23, pp113–25.

Engel S (1995) *The Stories Children Tell*, Plenum, New York.

Everett D (2008) *Don't Sleep, There Are Snakes*, Profile Books, London.

Fiese B (1999) *The Stories That Families Tell: Narrative Coherence, Narrative Interaction and Relationship Beliefs* (Monographs of the Society for Research in Child Development, 64 (2), pp1–36), Wiley, Chichester.

Fiestas C & Pena E (2004) 'Narrative discourse in bilingual children: language and task effects', *Language, Speech & Hearing Services in Schools*, 35 (2), pp155–68.

Fox C (1993) *At the Very Edge of the Forest: The Influence of Literature on Storytelling by Children*, Cassell, London.

Grove N (ed) (2013) *Using Storytelling to Support Children and Adults with Special Needs: Transforming Lives Through Telling Tales*, Taylor & Francis, London.

Grove N & Tucker S (2003) *Narratives in Manual Sign by Children with Intellectual Impairments*, Von Tetzchner S & Grove N (eds), *New Developments in Augmentative and Alternative Communication*, Whurr Publishers, London, pp230–55.

Gutierrez Clellen V & Quinn R (1993) 'Assessing from diverse linguistic/cultural groups', *Language, Speech and Hearing Services in Schools*, 24, pp2–9.

Heal L & Sigelman C (1995) 'Response bias in interviews of individuals with limited mental ability', *Journal of Intellectual Disability Research*, 39, pp331–40.

Herman R, Grove N, Holmes S, Morgan G, Sutherland H & Woll B (2004) *Assessing BSL Development: Production Test (Narrative Skills)*, City University, London.

Hudson J & Shapiro L (1991) 'From knowing to telling: the development of children's scripts, stories and personal narratives', McCabe A & Peterson C (eds), *Developing Narrative Structure*, Lawrence Erlbaum Associates, Hillsdale, NJ, pp89–136.

Hudson J, Gebelt J, Haviland J & Bentivegna C (1992) 'Emotion and narrative structure in young children's personal accounts', *Journal of Narrative and Life History*, 2, pp129–50.

Hymes D (1981) 'In vain I tried to tell you', *Essays in Native Ethnopoetics,* University of Pennsylvania, Philadelphia.

Keen E (2004) 'Developing the personal event narratives of children with autistic spectrum disorders', unpublished BSc dissertation, City University.

Kelly K & Bailey A (2013) 'Becoming independent storytellers: modeling children's development of narrative macrostructure', *First Language*, 33, pp68–89.

Labov W (1972) *Language in the Inner City*, University of Pennsylvania Press, Philadelphia.

Labov W & Waletzky J (1967) 'Narrative analysis: oral versions of personal experience', Helm J (ed), *Essays on the Verbal and Visual Arts,* University of Washington Press, Seattle, pp12–44.

Liles B (1993) 'Narrative discourse in children with language disorders and children with normal language: a critical review of the literature', *Journal of Speech & Hearing Research*, 36, pp868–82.

Mandler J & Johnson N (1977) 'Remembrance of things parsed: story structure and recall', *Cognitive Psychology*, 9, pp111–51.

McCabe A & Bliss L (2003) *Patterns of Narrative Discourse: A Multicultural Lifespan Approach*, Pearson Education, Boston MA.

McCabe A & Peterson C (eds) (1991a) *Developing Narrative Structure*, Lawrence Erlbaum Associates, Hillsdale, NJ.

McCabe A & Peterson C (1991b) 'Getting the story: a longitudinal study of parental styles in eliciting narrative and developing narrative skill', McCabe A & Peterson C (eds), *Developing Narrative Structure*, Lawrence Erlbaum Associates, Hillsdale, NJ, pp217–53.

McCabe A, Bliss L, Barra G & Bennett M (2008) 'Comparison of personal versus fictional narratives of children with language impairment', *American Journal of Speech – Language Pathology*, 17, pp194–206.

McHutchison L (2006) 'A comparison of communicative functions used by staff toward people with intellectual disabilities who are verbal or preverbal', BSc dissertation, City University, London.

Miller P & Sperry L (1988) 'Early talk about the past: the origins of conversational stories of personal experience', *Journal of Child Language*, 15, pp293–315.

Musselwhite C (1990) Topic setting: Generic & specific strategies *Paper presented to the 4th Biennial ISAAC Conference, Stockholm, 13–16th August.*

Nelson K & Gruendel J (eds) (1986) *Event Knowledge: Structure and Function in Development*, Lawrence Erlbaum Associates, Hillsdale, NJ.

Nicolopoulou A (1997) 'Children and narratives: toward an interpretive and sociocultural approach', Bamberg M (ed), *Narrative Development: Six Approaches*, Lawrence Erlbaum Associates, Mahwah, NJ, pp179–216.

Nind M & Hewett D (2005) *Access to Communication: Developing the Basics of Communication with People with Severe Learning Difficulties through Intensive Interaction* (2nd edition), David Fulton, London.

Nippold M (2007) *Later Language Development: School-Age Children, Adolescents, and Young Adults* (3rd edition), Pro-Ed, Austin, TX.

Norrick N (2000) *Conversational Narrative in Everyday Talk*, John Benjamin, Amsterdam.

Paley V (1991) *The Boy Who Would Be a Helicopter: Use of Storytelling in the Classroom*, Harvard University Press, Cambridge, MA.

Peter M & Sherratt-Smith D (2001) *Developing Drama and Play for Children With Autistic Spectrum Disorders*, David Fulton, London.

Peterson C & McCabe A (1983) *Developmental Psycholinguistics: Three Ways of Looking at a Child's Narrative*, Plenum Press, New York.

Peterson C, Jesso B & McCabe A (1999) 'Encouraging narratives in preschoolers: an intervention study', *Journal of Child Language*, 26, pp49–67.

Pratt M & Fiese B (2004) 'Families, stories, and the life course: an ecological context', Pratt M & Fiese B (eds), *Family Stories and the Life Course: Across Time and Generations*, Lawrence Erlbaum Associates, Mahwah, NJ, pp1–24.

Preece A (1987) 'The range of narrative forms conversationally produced by young children', *Journal of Child Language*, 14, pp353–73.

Propp V (1968) [1928] *Morphology of the Folktale*, trans Scott L, University of Texas Press, Austin, TX.

Reilly J, Klima E & Bellugi U (1990) 'Once more with feeling: affect and language in atypical populations', *Development and Psychopathology*, 2, pp367–91.

Schick B, Marschark M & Spencer P (eds) (2006) *Advances in the Sign Language Development of Deaf Children*, Oxford University Press, New York.

Scollon R (1979) 'A real early stage: an unzipped condensation of a dissertation on child language', Ochs E & Schieffelin B (eds), *Developmental Pragmatics*, Academic Press, New York.

Stein N & Albro E (1997) 'Building complexity and coherence: children's use of goal-sructured knowledge in telling stories', Bamberg M (ed) *Narrative Development: Six Approaches*, Lawrence Erlbaum Associates, Mahwah, NJ, pp5–44.

Tulving E & Craik F (2000) *The Oxford Handbook of Memory*, Oxford University Press, New York.

Turner M (1996) *The Literary Mind: The Origins of Thought and Language*, Oxford University Press, Oxford.

Vygotsky L (1978) *Mind in Society: The Development of Higher Psychological Processes*, Harvard University Press, Cambridge, MA.

Weir R (1962) *Language in the Crib*, Mouton, The Hague.

Further resources

Allen M, Kertoy M, Sherblom J & Pettit J (1994) 'Children's narrative productions: a comparison of personal event and fictional stories', *Applied Psycholinguistics*,15, pp149–76.

Applebee A (1978) *The Child's Concept of Story*, University of Chicago Press, Chicago.

Brice Heath S (1982) 'What no bedtime story means: narrative skills at home and school', *Language and Society*, 11, pp49–76.

Bruner J (1990) *Acts of Meaning*, Cambridge University Press, Cambridge.

Courage M & Cowan N (2008) *The Development of Memory in Infancy and Childhood*, Taylor & Francis, London.

Daniels H, Wertsch J & Cole M (eds) (2007) *The Cambridge Companion to Vygotsky*, Cambridge University Press, Cambridge.

Fivush R, Hammond N, Harsch N, Singer N & Wolf A (1991) 'Content and consistency in young children's autobiographical recall', *Discourse Processes*, 14, pp373–88.

Grove N, Harwood N, Ross V (2010) 'Sharing stories of everyday life with adults and children who have severe/profound intellectual disabilities' Prasher V (ed) *Contemporary Issues in Intellectual Disabilities*, Nova Publishers, pp225-30.

Killick S & Thomas S (2008) *Telling Tales: Storytelling as Emotional Literacy*, Educational Printing Services, Blackburn.

Minami M (2002) *Culture Specific Language Styles: The Development of Oral Narrative and Literacy*, Multilingual Matters, Clevedon.

Nelson K (1986) 'Event knowledge and cognitive development', Nelson K & Gruendel J (eds), *Event Knowledge: Structure and Function in Development*, Lawrence Erlbaum Associates, Hillsdale, NJ, pp1–20.

Ochs E & Capps L (2001) *Living Narrative: Creating Lives in Everyday Storytelling*, Harvard University Press, Cambridge, MA.

Reese E (2002) 'Social factors in the development of autobiographical memory: the state of the art', *Social Development*, 11, pp124–42.

Rogoff B, Mistry J, Goncu A & Mosier C (1993) *Guided Participation in Cultural Activity by Toddlers and Caregivers* (Monographs of the Society for Research in Child Development, 58 (8)), Wiley, Chichester.

Somers M (1994) 'The narrative construction of identity: a relational and network approach', *Theory and Society*, 23, pp605–49.

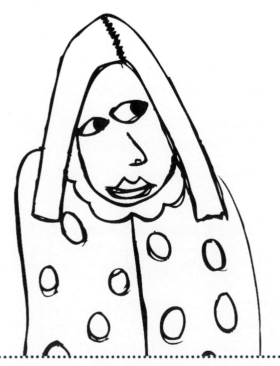

Speechmark ⑤

Theoretical background

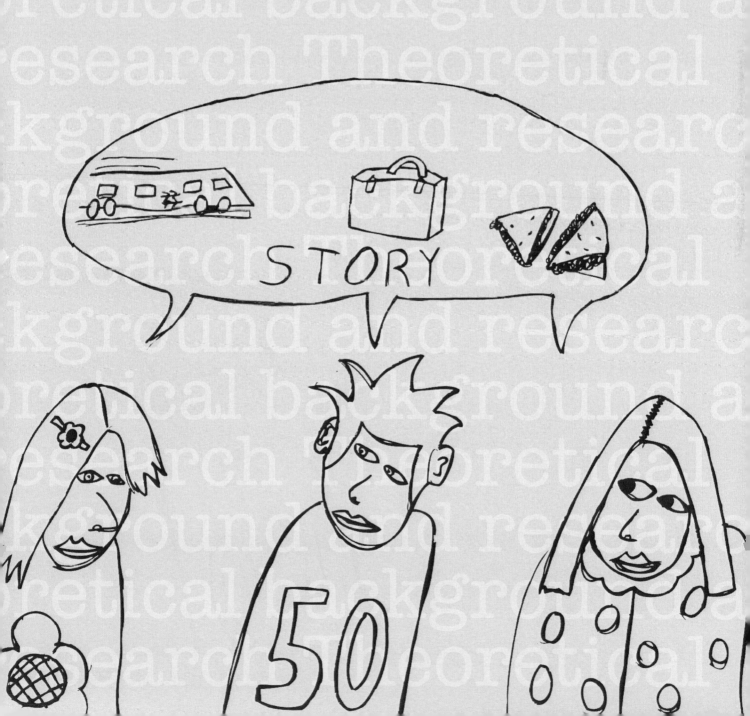

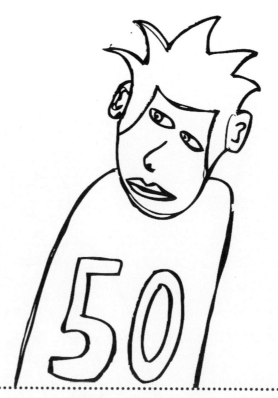

Speechmark

Introduction

Storysharing® was developed through a combination of practical experience, observation of anecdotal storytelling, and the study of different models of narrative. The theoretical framework is known as 'social constructionist', an approach to narrative that is associated mainly with the research of Carol Peterson, Alyssa McCabe and their collaborators. Another major influence was the groundbreaking research of Norrick (2000), who analysed the process in which anecdotes are created between adult narrators.

Theory and practice

One of the problems about the dominance of the fictional written narrative in education has been that (a) personal narratives have been almost completely ignored and (b) the models used for fictional narratives are imposed inappropriately on all kinds of oral telling. I have tried to stress in this book that there is no *one* approach to narrative development – rather, you should think about what you are trying to do, and what different approaches have to offer. The theory is really important. A theory is nothing more than the set of assumptions you are making when you work. The more you can understand about these assumptions, the better placed you will be to extend and adapt your work to real situations – especially when things don't go according to plan.

- How is narrative defined?
- Where do narratives come from?
- When do children start narrating?
- How does narrative develop in early childhood?
- How can we help children to become better narrators?[23]

Cognitive approaches: the story grammar model

This approach defines narrative as an account of causally related sequences of two or more events. The genesis of narrative is an inbuilt predisposition to see events as purposeful and causally linked. This structure influences a child's ability to remember events. As their memories and their ability to translate experience into language develops, so does their ability to narrate. The origin of storytelling, in this model, is mainly within the child's mind (*intrapersonal*). This means that children get better at narrating as they develop thinking skills. They start at around two and a half years, when they can put two events together in a sentence. During their third year, children begin to link events with *and* or *then*, but they don't include characters and settings until later. Not much happens under the age of about 4 (mental age equivalent, obviously). Of course, it is between 4 and 5 years that children are said to develop a 'theory of mind' (ie an understanding of motives and beliefs) and, from that time on, children begin to explore why characters behave in the way they do.

Narrative intervention within this model consists of helping children to include all of the relevant structural components in their narratives – using *wh-* questions, perhaps with colour coding, and reminding them to say who is involved, when and where the event happened, what happened (*at the beginning, then …, then …, at the end*).

Books and papers to look at if you are interested in the cognitive approach

Apparicio V, Shanks B & Rippon H (2007) *From Oral to Written Narrative*, Black Sheep Press, Keighley.

Stein N & Albro E (1997) 'Building complexity and coherence: children's use of goal-sructured knowledge in telling stories', Bamberg M (ed) *Narrative Development: Six Approaches*, Lawrence Erlbaum Associates, Mahwah, NJ, pp5–44.

Social process: the social constructionist model

A story is defined as an account of a reportable experience, involving a sequence of two or more events. Narratives emerge from a deep engagement and involvement in social interactions, as well as a cognitive predisposition to pay attention to what is novel and interesting, and to distinguish figure from ground. This underpins the subsequent cognitive development – which the social perspective does not ignore but sees as one dimension among many. The origins are seen as *interpersonal* as much as *intrapersonal*. Because narrative is a social process, it could be said to begin at birth.

Children develop as narrators as they express their feelings and respond to the feelings of others, take part in rhythmic repetitive games, and at about 9 months when they start to point out events of interest to other people. A baby sees something happen, looks at it, and turns to share it with someone else. They may point to it. Elizabeth Bates (1976) called these points-to-something-of-interest 'protodeclaratives', meaning that they were the foundations of the later language act of a statement or declarative. She firmly distinguished these kinds of points from communications which identified what children wanted – 'protoimperatives'. A paper by Ellis (2007) on preverbal narratives shows very clearly how this combination of an event noticed by the child, the suffusion of feelings, and their experience of rhythmic dialogue provides the underpinnings of oral narrative.

Social constructionists are interested in both the structural and the evaluative development of narrative. In terms of structure, they look for the kind of events that are expressed early on and the ways in which the climax or 'high point' of the story is expressed. Typically, children start with the most interesting event (the high point) and only later do they begin with initiating events and then move to a conclusion. For example, a child will come running in and say 'Knee! Fell down' at 2, and later 'I fell down and hurt my knee. Mummy put a plaster on it'.

These theorists broadly agree with the sequence of structural development outlined in the cognitive approach. There is not enough information as yet to set out in detail how children develop evaluation (the ability to express feelings, attitudes and judgements in story), but an early study has suggested that 3-year-olds may be more expressive narrators than 5-year-olds, perhaps because they are focusing less on all of the structural components (Reilly et al, 1990). Hudson and colleagues found that 4-year-olds produced highly expressive narratives relating to emotional experiences. Happy stories were told more to evoke mood, and were less structured than negative stories about anger and fear (Hudson et al, 1992).

With regard to intervention, the emphasis in the social model is on the way in which child narratives are scaffolded by the adults or older children who are involved in the conversation. *Scaffolding* is a term used to explain how adults and teachers will guide a child by supporting and extending their contributions.

Books and papers to look at for social constructionist approaches

Labov W & Waletzky J (1967) 'Narrative analysis: oral versions of personal experience', Helm J (ed) *Essays on the Verbal and Visual Arts,* University of Washington Press, Seattle, pp 12–44.

McCabe A & Bliss L (2003) *Patterns of Narrative Discourse: A Multicultural Lifespan Approach*, Pearson Education, Boston MA.

McCabe A & Peterson C (eds) (1991) *Developing Narrative Structure*, Lawrence Erlbaum Associates, Hillsdale, NJ.

Peterson C & McCabe A (1983) *Developmental Psycholinguistics: Three Ways of Looking at a Child's Narrative*, Plenum Press, New York.

Note

23 This set of questions is adapted from Michael Bamberg's book (1997), which compares different approaches to narrative development.

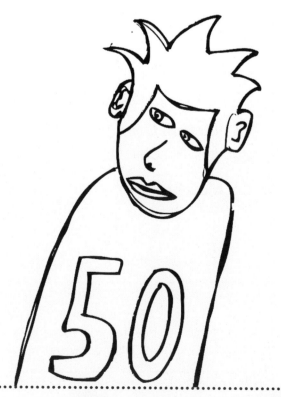

Examples of story records

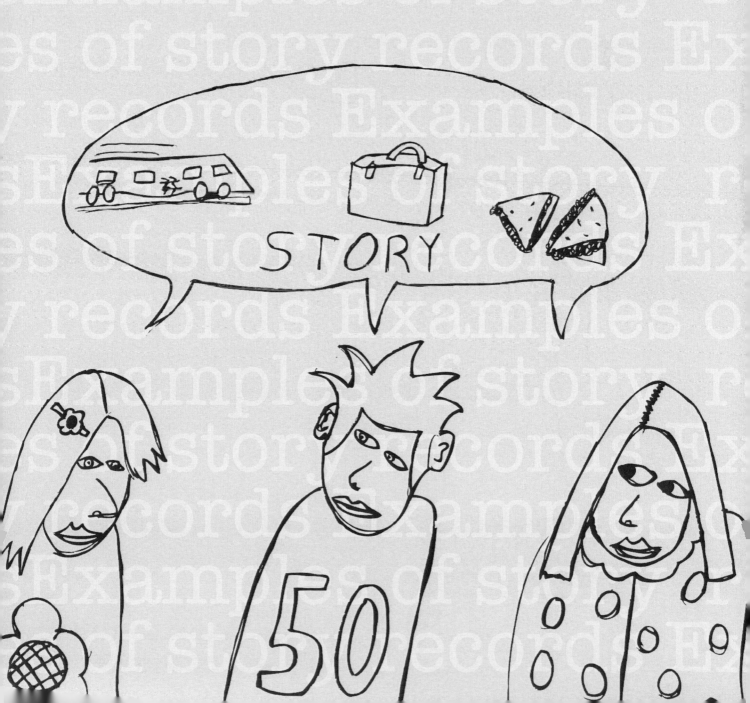

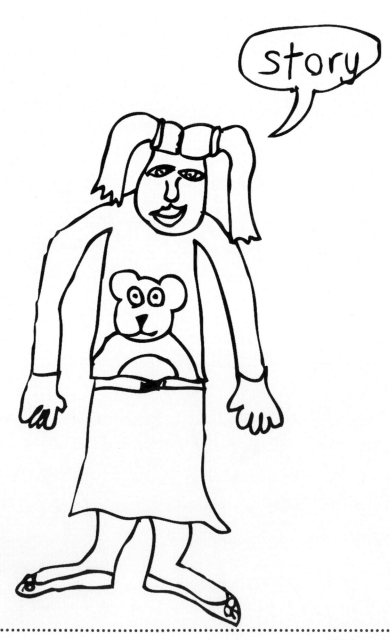

Speechmark

Introduction

These are some examples of ways in which stories could be recorded. Note, they are just ways of getting down the key information – you don't read through them out loud to tell the story. The first example is very linear and could be on one page of a scrapbook with a remnant on the other page. The second is more interactive – you can make a big picture of it and use sticky notes, then take a photograph of it. The third is a simple form which staff found it easiest to use to record not only what happened in the story, but also how it was told. You can laminate them as cards, or make them into books. Finally, there are some illustrations of more dynamic approaches – talking photo albums, puppets and memory boxes.

Story of the Week

What happened?

When & Where did it happen? -------------------------------------

----

Who was there? ---

What was said? ---

How did you feel? (*tick one or add your own..........*)

great   funny surprised excited proud frightened cross   sad embarrassed worried   ....

What did you 👁 --------------------

What did you 👂 --------------------

What did you 👃 -------------------

What did you 👂 -------------------

What did you 👄 -------------------

Anything else? ---

Write or draw some more about your story here. You could stick on something you found that reminds you of the story

---

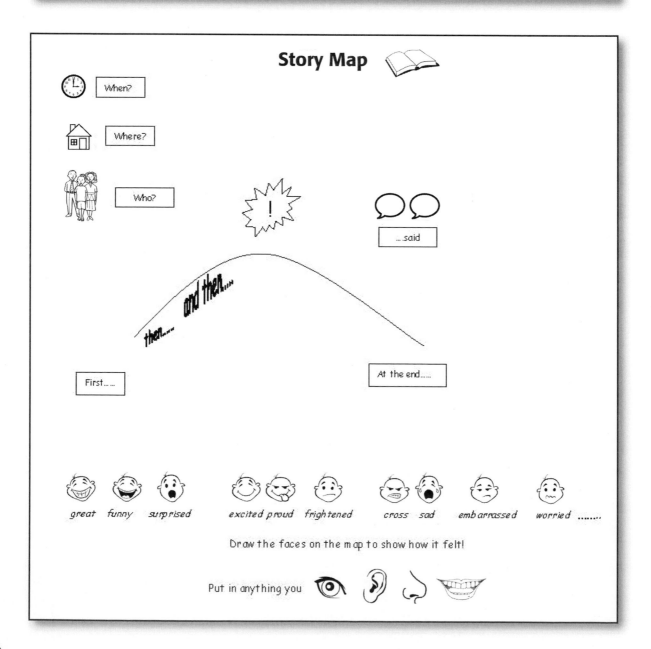

Story Map 📖

⏰ | When?

🏠 | Where?

👥 | Who?

...said

First.....

At the end......

great funny surprised   excited proud frightened   cross sad   embarrassed   worried ....

Draw the faces on the map to show how it felt!

Put in anything you 👁 👂 👃 👄

Story record form

The name of this story is _____

This story is told by _____

Write the story here	What do you say when telling the story?	How will the child respond? Note gestures, facial expressions, sounds, use of props as well as what she or he will say

What props do you use in the story?	How did it go? Add ideas for next time	Anything else?

Date: _____ Signed: _____

Story puppets

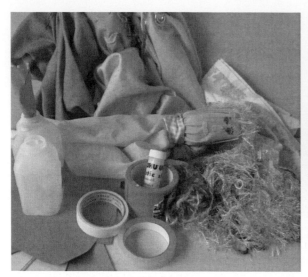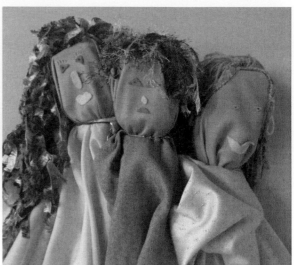

You need: a plastic milk bottle, a cloth, rubber bands and wooden spoons, plus materials to decorate.

Put a neutral colour cloth over the bottle for the puppet's head. Turn it upside-down.

Cut a hole in the middle of a square of cloth, and fasten it round the neck of the bottle.

Now you have a head and body. Insert a wooden spoon into the cavity to move the puppet. Decorate the face and add hair.

Stories can be written on slips of paper and placed in the 'head' of the puppet.

Thanks to Kate Burns (www.can-communicate.co.uk)

Memory boxes

Make a special box and decorate it: keep mementoes or treasured objects that tell a story inside it. This one has pictures of the houses where we lived, and was made by Derek Steele for my husband's 50th birthday.

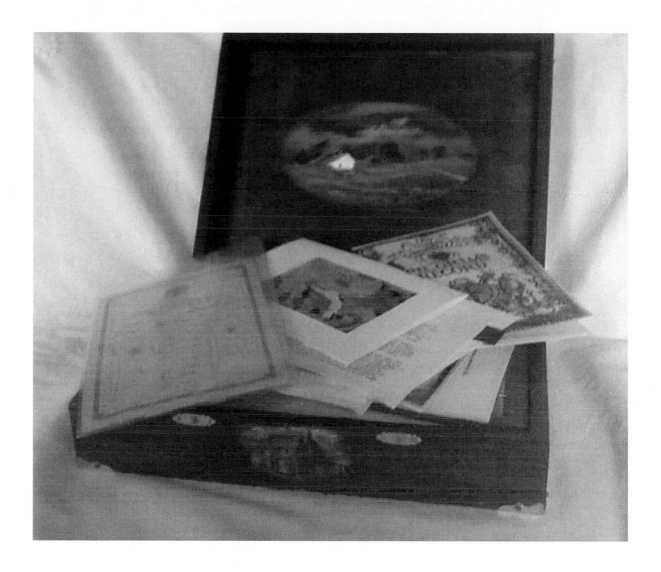

This is one of Kate Burns' boxes, with a collection of objects that are interesting to feel and handle, as well as being associated with stories.

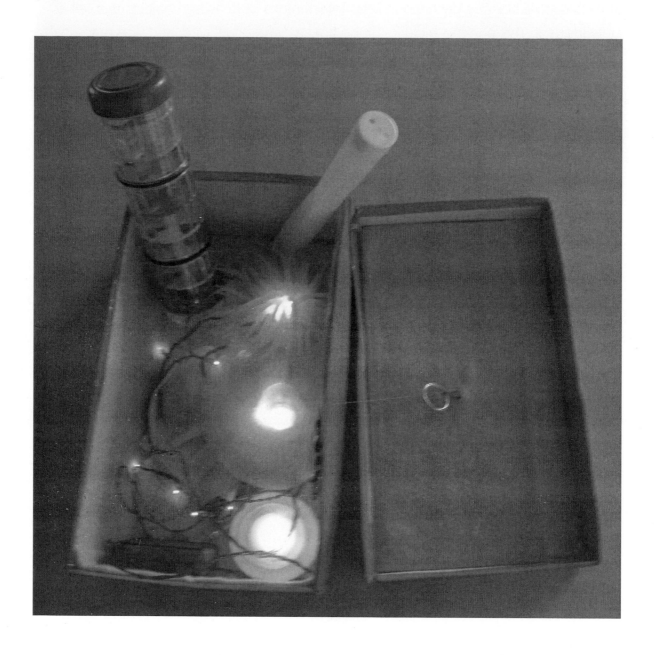

Story boxes and story puppets from an original idea by Kate Burns.
www.can-communicate.co.uk

Talking photo albums

The album has inserts in which you can put not only photos but also mementoes, clippings and newspaper articles. You record a message on a small recording button for each page. Messages can also be re-recorded.

A range of products can be found on the internet. There are also talking photo apps which will turn a portrait photo into a moving, speaking image.

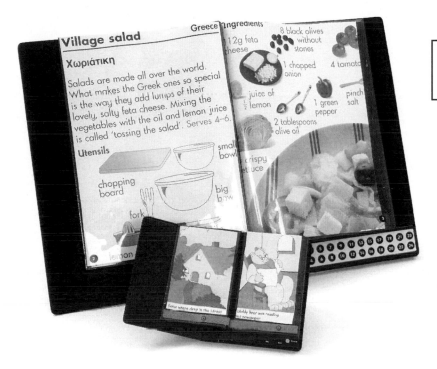

Talking photo album from Ablenet

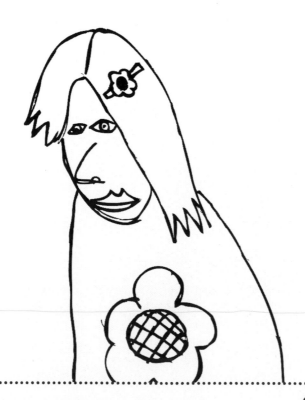

  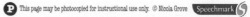

Assessment protocol

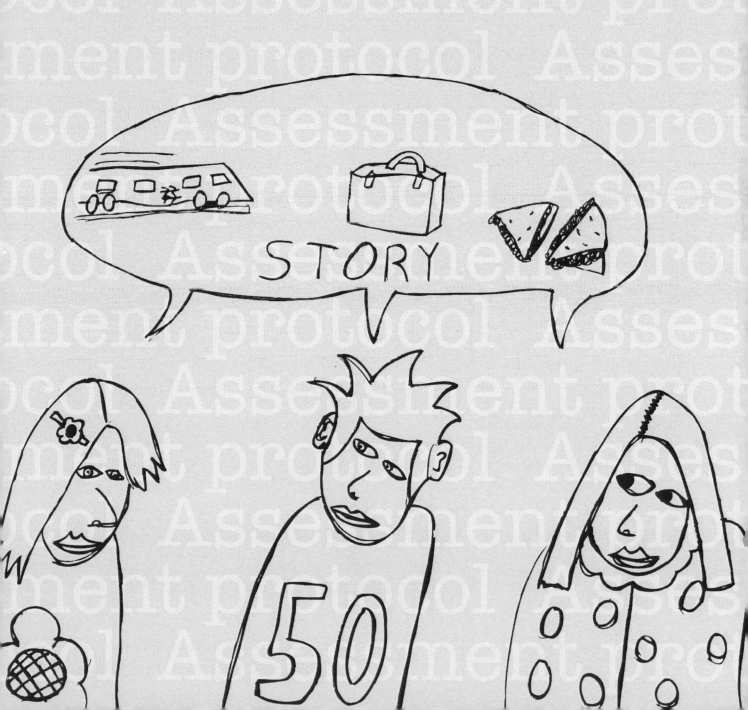

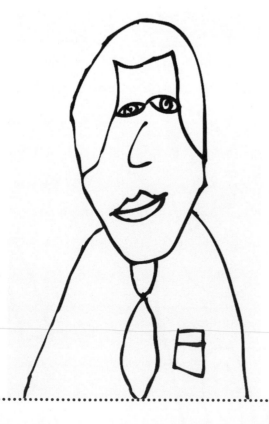

Introduction

We are going to tell some different kinds of stories – first, something just about what you do in the week, then stories about things that have happened in your life; first something negative or bad and then something really nice. The next one is a fairy story – can you remember a story you enjoyed when you were little? (Give examples if necessary.) And last, you get the chance to make up your very own story.

Scripts (narrative sequences about routines)

Tell me what you do during the week

Pick one or two events that are likely to involve well-known sequences of actions.

Tell me all about what happens when you …

Personal narratives: (a) negative, (b) positive

Can you remember a time when something not very nice or bad happened?

Maybe a time when you were scared, or angry or fed up?

Maybe something that happened when you were little, or something recent, like last week?

Can you remember a time when something really nice or funny happened?

Maybe a time when you were really happy, or which made you laugh?

Maybe something that happened when you were little, or something recent like last week?

Troubleshooting

Give positive feedback: *mm, yes, wow, oh no.*

Prompt with *and then?* if people get stuck.

If people come to a full stop, repeat what they said and ask *And what happens/ed then?*

End with positive affirmation of what the person has said.

If necessary, tell a short story of the appropriate genre yourself, to give them an idea. Ask: *Has anything like that ever happened to you?*

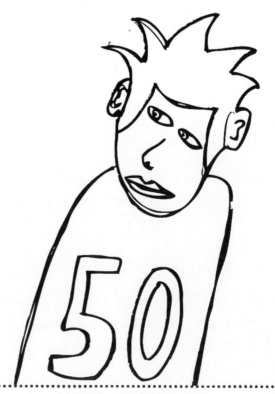

Speechmark

APPENDIX 4

Examples of stories told in different ways

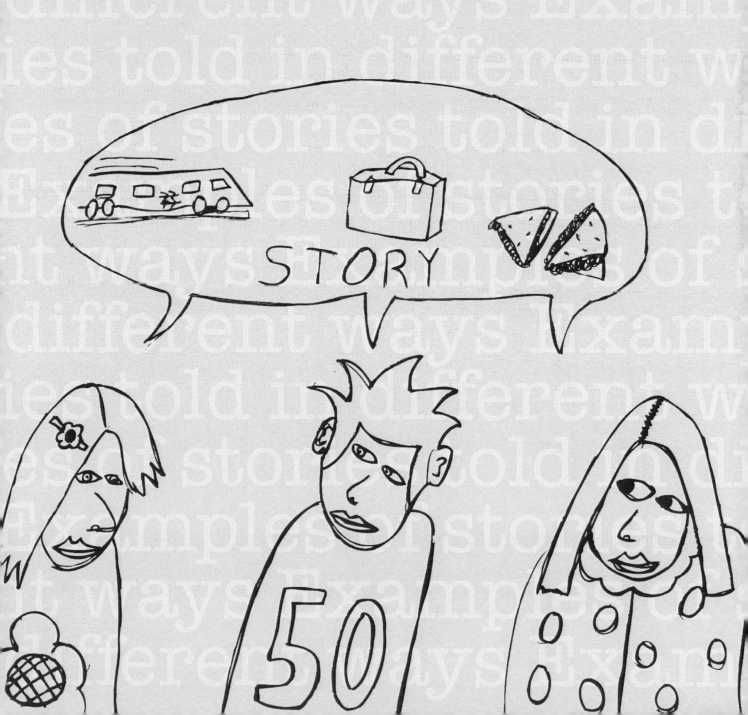

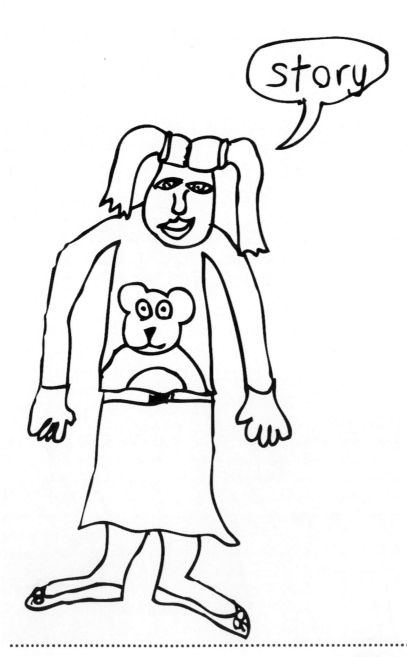

A story told by a group of children

Don't sleep in school!

A: [communication aid] This is what happened yesterday.

B: Holds up written sign TUESDAY.

A: [communication aid] It was really hot.

C: [verbal] We had to water the plants.

A: So Mrs Smith took the watering can.

D: (Holds up watering can.)

A: (She went outside.)

B: Shows clock.

A: She was a long time.

C: We went to look for her.

A: When we found her, guess what she was doing?

E: (Presses switch to make snoring sound.)

('Everyone laughs.)

Teacher: Guess what we did to wake her up?

Listener: You didn't!

Teacher and C: Yes we did (other children laugh and vocalise).

She got wet!

A story told by an adult supporting a child

Mowing the grass

Teacher: At the weekend, David and Mama and Papa were in the garden. And David was helping to cut the grass with the …

David: Lawn …

Teacher: Mower.

When suddenly …

David rises up in his chair with surprised expression, and throws his arms outwards. It is obvious what happened to the mower.

Teacher: It blew up! And mum said 'Oh well, another trip to B&Q.'

(Thanks to Corseford school for these stories)

A story told by mainstream and special school children working together

A story which emphasises rhythm and small achievements

Colin the wonder walker

(Make sound of walking.)

This term, Colin has been working really hard at walking and he has been walking and standing more and more, which is brilliant!

Every morning Colin has his leg gaiters put on and then he holds onto the walker and walks with Big Steve from Family Group 1 to the classroom.

Everyone walk to the chant:

Colin walked and he walked and he walked and he stopped

Colin walked and he walked and he walked and he stopped

Colin walked and he walked and he walked and he stopped

All the way to class until his legs went STOP!

Sometimes Colin really doesn't feel like walking and he will shout a lot, but once he has started walking, he stops shouting!

When he gets to class, he sits in his new class chair, wearing his gaiters.

(Thanks to Liz Platt for this story)

APPENDIX 5

Storysharing® profile

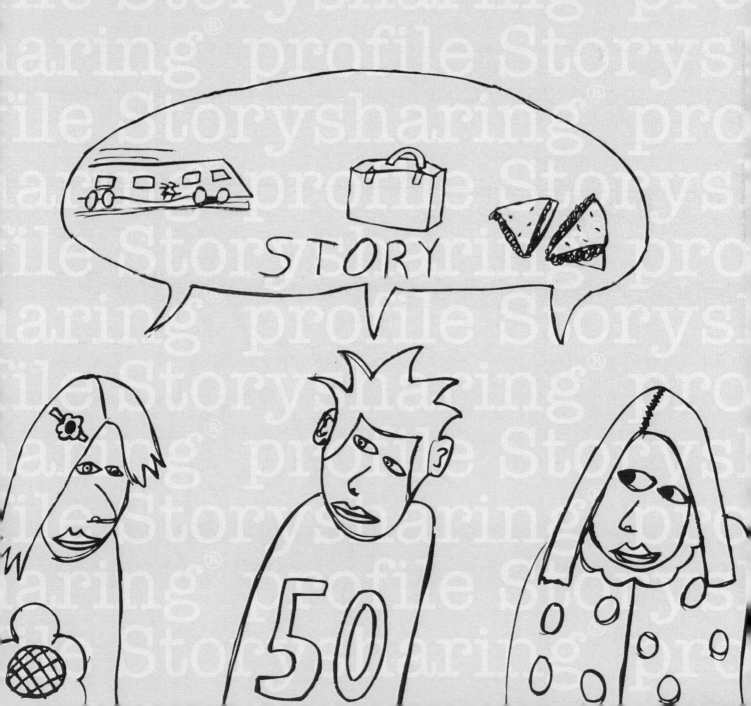

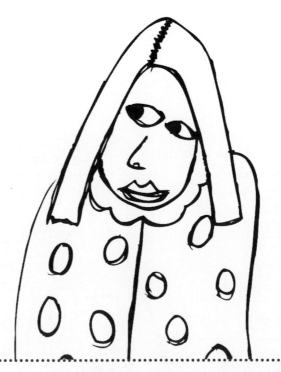

Speechmark

Skills for storytelling

Name: _____ **Date:** _____

Story type:

Story atmosphere: Funny/Sad/Happy/Exciting/Scary/Problem/Frustration/
Everyday routine/Other ...

Context:

Who is the story told to? Group/individual/naïve listener/informed listener

Story stimulus: Oral/Picture/Video/Other

Story outline: Provide a brief summary of the story told.

Collaboration and co-narration:

What is the balance of support and independent narration?

You can: count the number of 'turns' taken independently and with prompting by the
child which contribute to the narrative and express these as a proportion of the total.

You can: rate the amount of support needed, from 1(maximum) to 7 (minimal).

Comments:

What kind of support or prompt seems to help this child most?

Are any types of prompt unhelpful?

What kinds of contribution does the child seem to make independently? Eg gestures,
facial expressions, stock phrases, names of people, signs for actions.

At which points does the child join in?

Other comments

Skill	Observed	Comments
Social		
Beginning Ending		
Eye contact		
Audience awareness, eg pausing, repetition, response to questions		
Feeling and perspectives		
Gesture Mime Facial expression		
Reported speech Emotion words Judgements Mental state words		
Story structure		
Setting Participants Time Place Other (eg conditions)		
Actions Complicating actions High point Resolutions		

Skill	Observed	Comments
Recall and organisation of information		
Key information (*note how many events*) Sequencing (*note order correct or incorrect*)		
Language		
Vocabulary Nouns Adjectives Adverbs Verbs		
Sentence structure (*words or signs per sentence*)		
Poetic		
Intonation Stress Elongation Repetition Simile/metaphor Onomatopoeia Exaggeration		
Conventional phrases and sayings		
Reported speech Story language and conventions		

Skill	Observed	Comments
Listening		
Sits		
Allows physical prompt		
Orientates body		
Looks at teller		
Laughs		
Imitates sound		
Imitates movement		
Shows interest		
Recognition/recall		
Leans forwards		
Co-active gestures		
Reaches out		
Joins in		
Nods/shakes head in answer		
Gives feedback		
Answers questions		
Asks questions		
Comments		
Co-narrates		
Tells 'response' story		

Ideas for development

1 Identify what the main strengths and needs are for the child

Strengths in storytelling	Needs to develop

2 Identify what types of support help the child to tell stories

Prompts that help

Stimuli/resources that help

Who, when, where helps

3 Identify what the main focus of the intervention should be and one or two strategies for development

Focus	Strategies
Audience awareness	
Story structure	
Feeling and evaluation	
Recall and sequencing	
Language	
Listening	